GETTING PREGNANT
& STAYING PREGNANT

———————O

"This book is presented as a resource for women experiencing infertility and high-risk pregnancy. While it certainly meets this objective beautifully, the book is also an excellent reference for anyone contemplating, attempting, or experiencing pregnancy.

Diana Raab, the author, a nurse who has herself experienced infertility and two high-risk pregnancies, deals especially well with controversial topics such as vaginal birth after cesarean, commenting that it is both a personal and a professional decision. Throughout the book, there is sensitive discussion of the emotional aspects of everything from bed rest to Sudden Infant Death Syndrome.

Health care workers of all disciplines would do well to recommend this thorough and well-written book to women who want or need to know everything they can about getting or staying pregnant."

—Maternal Child Nursing

"An excellent information source on the complex issues and decisions of infertility and high-risk pregnancy. . . . The text well evokes the emotional impact on both partners, as well as the scientific aspects of these problems. . . . This well-illustrated book emphasizes the need for proper prenatal care and the importance of the prevention of problems before they arise."

—Booklist

"As a busy practicing obstetrician, I found the book *Getting Pregnant and Staying Pregnant* an extremely useful communication tool for the doctor and his staff and the high-risk OB patient. The book is well written in simple terminology, very practical and most of all comes from the heart and mind of a woman that was a patient herself. . . ."

—Katukota Vijay, M.D.
Obstetrics and Gynecology
Pomona Valley Medical Center

ORDERING

Trade bookstores in the U.S. and Canada please contact:

Publishers Group West
1700 Fourth Street, Berkeley, CA 94710
Phone: (800) 788-3123   Fax: (510) 528-3444

Hunter House books are available at bulk discounts
for textbook course adoptions; to qualifying community,
healthcare, and government organizations; and for special
promotions and fundraising. For details please contact:
Special Sales Department,
Hunter House Inc., PO Box 2914, Alameda, CA 94501-0914
Phone: (510) 865-5282 Fax: (510) 865-4295
e-mail: marketing@hunterhouse.com

Individuals can order our books from most bookstores
or by calling toll-free:
1-800-266-5592

GETTING PREGNANT & STAYING PREGNANT

—————— O ——————

Overcoming Infertility and Managing Your High-Risk Pregnancy

THIRD EDITION

DIANA RAAB, B.S., R.N.

Third edition revisions by
Anita Levine-Goldberg, RNP, MSN

Hunter House
PUBLISHERS

Hunter House Inc., Publishers
P.O. Box 2914
Alameda CA 94501-0914

Acknowledgment is made for permission to reprint: Poem on p. 41 from Centering Corporation; "Passive Exercises for Bedrest" (p. 154), adapted from the Good Samaritan Medical Center, Phoenix, Arizona; "Please Don't Tell Them You Never Got to Know Me" (p. 176) by Pat Schwiebert in *When Hello Means Goodbye* by P. Schwiebert and P. Kirk; "Popcorn and Waves" (p. 179) by Debbie Schleigh from *Unite Notes*, Unite Inc., 7600 Central Avenue, Philadelphia, PA 19111 © 1987; "The Sitting Time" (p. 187) by Joe Digman from *When Hello Means Goodbye* by P. Schwiebert and P. Kirk; "My Son" (pp. 227–229) by J.B. Bunnell, from *Neonatal Network*, © December 1986; chart (p. 241) from "Down's Syndrome and Maternal Age," adapted from J.A. Roberts, and M. Pembray, *An Introduction to Genetics*, Oxford University Press, 1985; "Internal Female Reproductive Anatomy" illustration (p. 268) and "Fertilization and Implantation of the Egg" illustration (p. 271) from *The Fertility Awareness Workbook* by B. Kass-Annese, R.N. and H.C. Danzer, M.D., Hunter House, 1989.

Library of Congress Cataloging-in-Publication Data
Raab, Diana, 1954–
Getting pregnant and staying pregnant : overcoming infertility
and managing your high-risk pregnancy / Diana Raab. — Rev. ed.
p. cm.
Previously published in 1991.
Includes bibliographical references and index.
ISBN 0-89793-238-2
1. Infertilit—Popular works. 2. Pregnancy—Complications—Popular works. I. Title.
RG201.R33   1999
618.1'78-dc21   99-26874
CIP

Project credits
Cover Design: Ame Beanland   Book Production: Andrea Reider
Copy Editor: Rosana Francescato   Project Editor: Jennifer Rader
Third Edition Revisions: Anita Levine-Goldberg, Jennifer Rader
Managing Editor: Wendy Low   Illustrations: Norma Dvorsky-Couture
Acquisitions Coordinator: Jeanne Brondino
Proofreader: Lee Rappold   Indexer: Kathy Talley-Jones
Publicity: Marisa Spatafore
Customer Service Manager: Christina Sverdrup
Order Fulfillment: Joel Irons, A & A Quality Shipping Services
Publisher: Kiran S. Rana

Printed and Bound by Bang Printing, Brainerd, Minnesota
Manufactured in the United States of America

9 8 7 6 5 4 3   Third Edition   05 06 07 08 09

Contents

———O———

Foreword

———————O———————

As an obstetrician specializing in high-risk pregnancies, I understand the possible dangers and obstacles associated with pregnancy. Many couples have a hard time becoming pregnant and carrying their baby to full term, and all couples need to understand what is necessary for a successful pregnancy as well as the potential risks. This book provides an excellent resource to help couples understand important pregnancy issues such as infertility, high-risk complications, birth defects, and genetic risks.

Getting Pregnant and Staying Pregnant provides a clear and concise dialogue on the causes of infertility as well as what can be expected of a high-risk pregnancy. Many tests and procedures are clearly defined, enabling the expectant couple to be very well prepared. This book discusses the causes of high-risk pregnancy and offers some solutions to help couples deal with such a fragile time.

It is crucial for couples to be well informed about the possible complications as well as the possible successful outcomes of a full-term pregnancy. Diana Raab does a tremendous job of providing readers with an easy-to-read and easy-to-understand account of this special time in a woman's life. She also includes throughout the book anecdotes and stories from parents who have experienced the trials and tribulations of infertility and miscarriages, as well as stories detailing successful full-term pregnancies.

Getting Pregnant and Staying Pregnant is a compassionate book. It serves a wonderful purpose in describing what can happen in a high-risk pregnancy and what can be done to ensure that the pregnancy is carried through a full term.

— Harry Farb, M.D.
Director of Maternal-Fetal Medicine,
North Memorial Medical Center, Minneapolis, Minnesota
Clinical Associate Professor of Obstetrics and Gynecology,
University of Minnesota, Department of OB/GYN

Acknowledgments

———————— O ————————

Anyone who has written a book knows about the joy and despair that accompany the experience. It is an endeavor that demands an enormous amount of love and devotion for the subject. It is a task that dominates the author's life until the day of completion. I am delighted that the new millennium will welcome the third edition of my book. The fact that there is still a demand for a book of this type is indicative that women continue to want to be informed about their bodies and that the issues remain the same.

Yet a book of this kind is rarely, if ever, written alone. Numerous people who cross the path of the author during the writing of a book affect its final form. From the day this book was conceived nearly sixteen years ago, I owe much to many people who have offered their comments and criticism during the preparation of the original manuscript. In particular, I wish to acknowledge Andrew Mok, M.D., for his dedicated commitment to being available when we needed him during all three of my difficult pregnancies and for his valuable review of the manuscript in its early stages.

Others who helped greatly with this book are:

James E. Clark, M.D., Hal C. Danzer, M.D., Alan H. DeCherney, M.D., Frederick Hoover, M.D., George Huggins, M.D., Barbara Kass-Annese, R.N., C.N.P., Mary Kostenbauder, M.S.N., R.N., Mehrnaz Sajedi, R.D., and Ed Siegall, M.D.

And

Norma Dvorsky-Couture, who believed in this project as much as I did, Barbara Provan, a dear friend who brought me lunch every day of bed rest during my first pregnancy, Dennis Gross, M.D., my kids' pediatrician, and my beloved mentor, Lynda Percival Glickman, R.N., whose friendship I will miss forever.

And

Kiran Rana, my publisher, who nearly ten years ago saw the value of my book and bought the rights after I had self-published it three years prior, and the staff at Hunter House, especially Jennifer Rader. A special thanks to Anita Levine-Goldberg, who prepared the revisions for this third edition.

And

Rachel, Regine, and Joshua, my children, who gave me a kiss every time I went to the office to write the original manuscript and who now brag about the book to their friends; my mom, Eva Klein Marquise, for her encouragement; my beloved father, Ed Marquise, for all his love and adoration; my husband's parents, Jeannine and Alexandre, for their love and support throughout; and my grandparents, whom I wish my children could have known.

And

Most important, my husband, Simon, whose unfailing support, love, and encouragement helped me make it through three high-risk pregnancies and whose enthusiasm and technical support helped bring this project to fruition.

Diana Raab
Florida, 1999

IMPORTANT NOTE

The material in this book is intended to provide a review of information regarding infertility, high-risk pregnancy, and delivery. Every effort has been made to provide accurate and dependable information. The contents of this book have been carefully reviewed by medical doctors. However, health care professionals have differing opinions and ways of treating various problems, and advances in medical and scientific research are made very quickly, so that some of the information may become outdated.

Therefore, the publisher, author, editors, and reviewers cannot be held responsible for any error, omission, or dated material. Any of the treatments described should be undertaken only under the guidance of a licensed health-care practitioner. The author and publisher assume no responsibility for any outcome of the use of any of these treatments in a program of self-care or under the care of a licensed practitioner.

If you have a question concerning your care or treatment, or about the appropriateness or application of the treatments described this book, consult your health-care professional.

Introduction: My Story

This book began as a diary of my five months of bed rest during my first pregnancy and then progressed to include information and the experiences of other women. Now, in its final form, it is a guide for and about women who are having trouble conceiving and/or are having difficult pregnancies.

Although a nurse, I was eager for more information when I became pregnant. Friends and colleagues would bring me books about normal pregnancy and I felt as if I never fit into any of the categories described. I was not having a normal pregnancy. That is why I decided to write this book. I hope that if women understand what is happening inside of them they will gain confidence in themselves, what they are going through, and the decisions they make. Many of the women I interviewed for the anecdotes in this book told me that my book has taken the mystery out of their problems. Often, our imagination is much worse than reality.

High-risk pregnancies are not fun. They seem to drag on forever. By sharing my story with you, I hope I can help you see the light at the end of the tunnel. Today, my husband and I have three healthy children, two daughters and a son—the happy ending to this story. But reaching this point was far from easy.

My husband and I are both career professionals and worked for five years after we got married before deciding to start a family. Pregnancy was not an easy task for us. It took me over a year to become pregnant. When I found out I was pregnant I was ecstatic, and just like many inexperienced mothers-to-be, I saw no harm in spreading the good news. Within the first two months I was dressing in maternity clothes. Unfortunately, my enthusiasm was shattered by a miscarriage at only twelve weeks.

My obstetrician was away the weekend I miscarried and was very surprised the following Monday morning when I told him the news. It was all the more shocking for us because that past Friday we had heard the baby's heartbeat during my routine prenatal visit, and everything seemed perfect.

It took me a very long time to accept our loss, and I found it particularly difficult when I saw other women with their own children. It seemed like a constant reminder of my failure. Over the next few months the cause of my miscarriage was investigated. The first test I had, a hysterosalpingogram, showed that I had a congenital uterine abnormality and a cervical condition, which meant that without proper intervention, I would be unable to carry a baby to term.

I learned that because of these congenital problems the only way I would be able to carry a baby to term was to have major surgery. Perhaps because I was a nurse, I was afraid to have the surgery. I was aware of all the things that could go wrong. I urged my obstetrician to take the most conservative approach. He told me that surgery was the only solution, and that if I were his wife he would make the same recommendation.

We sought a second opinion from an obstetrician specializing in this type of surgery. He also recommended surgery. I was still uncomfortable with the idea, and so I sought yet another opinion. The third obstetrician had a different philosophy, one closer to mine. He claimed that with each pregnancy my double uterus would become stretched and I would be able to carry a fetus longer each time until I eventually carried to term. I already knew that I would have to have a cervical suture early in my pregnancy to solve the problem of my inadequate or "incompetent cervix."

Nine months later I was pregnant. I was having problems right from the beginning of my pregnancy. Around my sixth week I began spotting. Because it was the weekend (somehow all my problems occurred on holidays or weekends), we went to my hospital's emergency department and were told that there are two possible reasons for spotting early in pregnancy—impending miscarriage or low progesterone levels.

Because of my history of hormonal imbalances, it was decided that I needed two progesterone injections spaced two weeks apart. My obstetrician said that if the spotting was indeed due to a defective egg, I would abort during that two-week period. Luckily, that didn't happen.

At twelve weeks, I was given a cervical suture to ensure that I would be able to carry my baby. I remained in the hospital for three days and was sent home on a medication to prevent premature contractions, which could have put the suture under stress. I took these pills for the remainder of my pregnancy.

Unfortunately, because the suture was inserted after my cervix had begun dilating, I had to stay in bed for five months. I was tempted to write Sophia Loren, who underwent the same ordeal. Because I really wanted that baby, I did everything my obstetrician recommended. I was advised not to climb stairs, and as a result had to stay on the upper level of our two-story home.

Each day was full of surprises. I had mild contractions a few times daily and visited the emergency unit, as it turned out, once a month for the next five months. I spotted throughout the pregnancy and was told that my suture was being stressed and that I should take it easy. I never knew how long I would carry my baby. In my husband's words, every day was another blessing! It's impossible to describe the paradoxical passage of time—those days in bed that passed so quickly, yet also seemed to drag on for eternity. I can't even begin to catalogue my emotions, which seemed to ricochet off the bedroom walls for those five long months.

Finally, at thirty-two weeks, approximately four weeks short of what is known as "the term of pregnancy," I gave birth by cesarean to a beautiful 4½-pound baby girl. Although she didn't cry at birth and was completely blue, it was the happiest moment of my life. Her first few moments of oxygen support were enough to give her the strength to carry on a life of her own.

The next happiest day of my life was two years later to the day, when I gave birth again, this time to a perfect 8-pound girl, who I have been told could have been in baby commercials. This second pregnancy was much easier, partly because I knew what to expect. My husband and I breathed a sigh of relief knowing that this baby was not premature—she was a very strong and healthy baby.

And at last, three years later, I gave birth to my one and only son. This was an easier pregnancy. I was much more active and confident that all would go well—and it did.

○

The purpose of this book is to provide women and concerned health professionals with a guide to infertility and difficult pregnancies. I offer some tips and suggestions on issues that I have not seen addressed in other related books. And I hope the quotes from mothers I interviewed will show the infertile couple and high-risk mother that they are not alone.

Those readers who feel they would benefit from an overview of the male and female reproductive anatomy should refer to Appendix A. Having a clear understanding of how the body works will help you in your interactions with caregivers and medical specialists. Appendix B is an extensive list of support groups, organizations, and information sources that will be helpful for mothers and couples who are facing the concerns and issues discussed in the book. There is also a glossary to explain any medical or technical terms.

While sharing my knowledge is important, I feel I can offer special encouragement and support because I have been there. I have experienced the needs, the joys, the sorrows, the pains, and worst of all, the uncertainties. And still, although all three of my pregnancies were difficult physically and emotionally, sixteen years after my first pregnancy, all the problems I had seem insignificant now, as I watch my three children blossom into beautiful young adults. I realize that every difficult moment I had to undergo for them to be born was something I wouldn't have missed for anything in the world!

Chapter 1

———————— O ————————

Causes of Infertility

Infertility is defined as the inability to become pregnant after one year of sexual intercourse with no contraceptive protection. Those couples trying to have children consider it a tragedy unlike any other in their lives. The infertile couple may be laden with fears, stresses, concerns, and questions that often only careful medical evaluation can address. It is normal to feel depressed and discouraged as plans for parenthood seem to drift into the nebulous future.

Nearly 20 percent of all couples trying to become pregnant are affected by infertility. In about 30 to 40 percent of those cases, the cause of infertility is related to the woman; in another 10 to 30 percent it is related to the man; 15 to 30 percent of the time it is related to problems involving both the male and female partners; and in another 10 to 15 percent it is unexplained.

In both men and women, infertility may be caused by a combination of anatomical/physiological problems, hormonal imbalances, genetic alterations, exercise/nutritional habits, certain prescription and illicit drugs, environmental hazards, and emotional factors.

CAUSES OF MALE INFERTILITY

Low Sperm Count

Oligospermia, or low sperm count, is the primary cause of male infertility. Many sperm are killed by normal vaginal secretions or lost during their journey to the fallopian tubes. A man who begins with a lower-than-usual sperm count may find he has an infertility problem. Normally, sixty million or more sperm per cubic centimeter are delivered with each ejaculation in a volume ranging from one to four cubic centimeters of semen.

Actual sperm production may be influenced by anatomical conditions, hormones, nutrition, environmental pollutants, industrial chemicals, marijuana, radiation exposure, or certain illnesses. Certain medications, such as large doses of aspirin, Cimetidine (used to treat duodenal ulcers), and Nitrofurantoin (antibacterial medication), may also affect fertility. Diethylstilbestrol (DES), the synthetic female hormone prescribed for many pregnant women to prevent miscarriage between 1941 and 1971, has been associated with male infertility: sons of women who have taken this drug have been found to have abnormal sperm type and motility in addition to testicle abnormalities. You should alert your specialist if your partner has been exposed to DES. Your partner should also be advised to do monthly testicle examinations and to report any lump, growth, or swelling to a urologist. Researchers report that crash diets also have a tendency to lower sperm count, just as strict diets can lead to irregular menstrual cycles in women.

It is now known that warmer temperatures may also hinder sperm production. Some researchers suggest that taking saunas and hot baths can cause overly high temperatures in the scrotal sac, an effect that may hinder sperm production for months. Men who wear tight clothing may be lowering their sperm count as well. Often, males with infertility problems are advised not to wear tight-fitting pants or underwear.

Oligospermia is sometimes treated with Clomid or Humagon. In the United States, Clomid and Humagon have not been approved by the Food and Drug Administration for treating male infertility, so in many cases the male must sign a special consent form prior to beginning the treatment.

In some cases, steroids, antiprostaglandins, or vitamins C and E are recommended to increase sperm count. A study reported in the *Journal of the American Medical Association* in 1983 by Dr. Earl Dawson at the University of Texas Medical Center showed that a daily dosage of vitamin C may restore fertility. The men in the study were given a one-month supply of vitamin C in 500 mg gelatin capsules. One tablet was to be taken every twelve hours. It was concluded that the men's fertility could be restored as early as the third or fourth day of treatment. Other studies have shown that an increased intake of zinc and vitamin E may also increase sperm count. These treatments and similar ones remain controversial and should be undertaken only under careful medical supervision.

Anatomical Changes

The tubes, or ducts, that carry the sperm may have flaws that affect fertility. This is the problem for approximately 10 percent of infertile men. Studies indicate that this flaw—often caused by a blockage—is more evident in men whose mothers took DES and among men who have had genital infections or surgery.

The spermatic cord is the cord suspending the testes. It is composed of veins, arteries, lymphatics, nerves, and the vas deferens, which carries the sperm from the epididymis to the ejaculatory duct (see the diagram Male Reproductive Anatomy in Appendix A).

A varicocele is an enlargement of the veins of the spermatic cord. It affects fertility by producing a slightly higher temperature in the testicles, which hinders sperm production. It is present in about 15 percent of all men, usually on the left side, and it accounts for about 40 percent of male infertility problems. As many as 90 percent of the men who have previously fathered a child and are later unable to have this problem.

Varicoceles are treated surgically. The success rate varies; it is estimated that approximately 80 percent of men have an increased sperm count following this surgery. The most common type of procedure is microsurgery, which is done on an outpatient basis under spinal anesthesia. The stitches are self-dissolving, and the man goes home with tiny Steri-Strips or Band-Aids to be removed in ten days. Some specialists prescribe fertility medications such as Clomid to stimulate sperm production following the surgery.

A scrotal injury may also cause male infertility, if the injury affects the blood supply and sperm transportation. Another cause of infertility may be an undescended testicle (corrected or uncorrected). The cool temperatures that allow sperm production are not possible if the testicle is hidden in the abdominal cavity. A male whose testicles descend late in life may also be prone to infertility, and yet an undescended testicle does not necessarily result in infertility problems.

Previous Illness

A history of certain infections, such as mumps, may be another cause of male infertility. If a male gets the mumps during or just after puberty, there is a risk that the virus will attack the testicles. In severe cases, the man will have an increased risk of infertility problems later in life. Sexually transmitted diseases, such as chlamydia, have also been linked to infertility and low sperm count.

Genetics and Hormonal Imbalances

In rare instances, infertility in the male may be inherited. This is usually identified through chromosomal tests. Treatment is often difficult unless the condition is related to a particular problem, such as hormonal deficiency, which can be treated with hormonal replacements. Hormonal problems account for approximately 10 to 15 percent of male infertility. Some imbalances may be due to a poorly functioning pituitary gland. Standard hormone analyses are not often done on the male, mainly because of their cost; an exception is if an abnormality was found in the semen analysis.

CAUSES OF FEMALE INFERTILITY

Ovulation Problems

The most common cause of female infertility is the failure to ovulate regularly or at all, which in turn is usually related to hormonal problems.

Common Reasons for Hormonal Imbalances

○ *Age.* The release of reproductive hormones diminishes after a woman's twenties, and therefore women will ovulate less often.

○ *Pituitary tumor.* This may inhibit the release of FSH and LH at the right time during the menstrual cycle, thereby affecting ovulation.

○ Pituitary gland problems. For example, one such problem is elevated levels of prolactin, the hormone that stimulates breast milk production and blocks ovulation.

O Adrenal gland problems. These cause increased levels of androgen, a hormone that interferes with ovulation.

Other causes of ovulation problems include disorders of the ovary, such as an ovarian cyst, overexercising, nutritional deficiencies, and certain medications.

Many practitioners claim that an abnormal menstrual history may be a clue that there is or will be an ovulation problem. By the age of fifteen or sixteen, the menstrual cycle should be more or less regular, with a menstrual period every twenty-eight days or so. If, however, the number of days between periods varies greatly, this may indicate a hormone regulation or timing problem associated with ovulation. This does not mean that if you have irregular periods you will have difficulty becoming pregnant. It means that if you have irregular periods there is a greater chance that you may ovulate late each month or maybe ovulate only every other month. One of my patients ovulated only twice each year.

For the most part, those women who get pregnant very easily are those who have very regular periods. Most women who do not ovulate on a regular basis have a slightly elevated level of male hormone. Signs of increased male hormone include extra facial hair, hair on the lower abdomen, hair on the big toe, and extra hair around the anus. Acne and oily skin may also be associated with excessive male hormone.

Older women who have used the birth control pill for many years may also find that ovulation is temporarily reduced or stopped. In most cases, the Pill does not affect a woman's fertility if she had normal menstrual cycles prior to starting the Pill. Those who stop taking the Pill and have difficulty getting pregnant may not have been ovulating spontaneously before. A medical investigation may be recommended if you have gone off the Pill and fail to have a normal menstrual cycle within five to six months.

Fertility Drugs

Your specialist will quickly identify ovulation problems through your temperature charts. If your temperature charts indicate that you are not ovulating, the specialist will probably prescribe a fertility drug, such as clomiphene (Clomid). Other fertility drugs include Humagon, GnRH, and Parlodel. These and related drugs are discussed in more detail below.

Clomiphene (Clomid)   Clomid is a synthetic drug that signals the pituitary gland to produce hormones that stimulate ovulation. It is used when the woman's ovaries and hormonal networks are capable of working well but simply need some "revving up." Even if the woman is menstruating irregularly, Clomid helps develop follicles that are not reaching their normal size and helps immature follicles grow to maturity. Approximately 75 to 80 percent of women will ovulate using this medication; however, the pregnancy rate is only about 30 to 40 percent. Those women who do not become pregnant usually go on to use Menotropins or ART.

The dosage of Clomid varies, but it usually begins with a 50 mg tablet daily starting on the third day of the menstrual cycle. If the woman does not ovulate during the first cycle, the dose may be doubled or eventually tripled. Women respond differently to Clomid and this is why an initial low dose is used. While taking Clomid, it is recommended that you continue with your temperature charts or ovulator predictor kit. The length of time required to produce results is highly individual, and sometimes it is necessary to have three courses of treatment to achieve results.

There is a risk of multiple births following the use of this drug and all other fertility medications. A twin pregnancy may occur in about one out of fifty women taking Clomid.

One woman shares her experience:

My lifelong desire to have children was fulfilled when I learned in my sixth month of pregnancy that I was having twins. I knew there would be the possibility, because there's a history of twins in my family, plus I had been on Clomid for four months.

Sometimes it takes longer for fertility medications to work, as this woman describes:

I thought when I popped my first fertility drug I'd be pregnant immediately; however, when four years later I was still not pregnant, it became a real mental strain. I began to think I'd never become pregnant. My treatments seemed to be never-ending. I tried various doses of Clomid, and then finally Humagon was my success drug. This is easy to say now, however, as I sit here with three children under the age of ten.

Some women experience mild side effects from the medication, such as water retention, hot flashes, visual disturbances, abdominal discomfort, and tender breasts. You should notify your physician if you have unusual bloating, stomach or pelvic pain, blurred vision, nausea/vomiting, or any other unusual symptoms.

Menotropins (Humagon, Fertinex) Depending upon your fertility problem, if you fail to ovulate in response to larger doses of clomiphene and have low estrogen levels, your specialist may recommend a stronger medication called human menopausal gonadotropin (hMG), more commonly known as Humagon. Humagon, formerly called Pergonal, belongs to a group of drugs called Menotropins. It contains natural, purified follicle-stimulating hormone (FSH) and luteinizing hormone (LH), and it may also be taken instead of Clomid. Developed in the 1960s, this medication stimulates the ovaries to ovulate and is usually given by injection for several days, beginning on the second or third day of the menstrual cycle. Prior to Humagon treatment you will have an ultrasound to be sure that you have no ovarian cysts; if there are large cysts, they will have to be removed prior to beginning this treatment.

Humagon is generally given under close daily supervision, including watching for cervical mucus changes, ovarian enlargement, and changing estrogen levels. When the eggs are mature, an injection of 10,000 IU of hMG is given and ovulation often occurs within thirty-six hours, at which time intercourse or intrauterine insemination is recommended.

Humagon tends to decrease progesterone levels. For this reason, you may need progesterone injections beginning two to five days after the Humagon. Progesterone is a hormone that is naturally produced by the body to allow the embryo to implant itself in the uterus.

Humagon is very expensive, and it is used only by qualified physicians who have easy access to ultrasound devices. The most significant side effect of this medication is the formation of ovarian cysts, which rarely have to be removed surgically. According to Facts and Comparisons, a drug information and publication service, approximately 80 percent of those taking Humagon will have single births; 15 percent will have twin births, and 5 percent will have three or more fetuses.

GnRH (Gonadotropin-Releasing Hormone) GnRH is produced by the hypothalamus and stimulates the pituitary gland to produce FSH and LH. This medication, sometimes known as Lutrepulse, is used when Clomid is ineffective. Some physicians prescribe it prior to Humagon, while others recommend it after Humagon has failed. Yet other specialists may choose to use these medications in combination.

Lutrepulse is given with a battery-operated pump held in a pocket with a tube leading to a vein in the arm. The medication is administered every ninety minutes until ovulation occurs, mimicking natural hormonal release. The technique is similar to that for diabetics receiving continuous doses of insulin and may be done in the hospital. Some women are now given the option of home administration by their partners. The dose and number of treatments vary with the individual; however, once the right dose is determined for you, you will probably respond to a similar dose in subsequent cycles.

According to Ortho Pharmaceuticals, the manufacturer of Lutrepulse, the treatment cycle is twenty-one days, and the cost is approximately $1,200 to $1,500. This cost includes the medication and pump, an ultrasound, and physician visits. Approximately 93 percent of those taking this medication will ovulate following the treatment, and about 62 percent will get pregnant. The actual dose is approximately 5 mcg every ninety minutes.

Parlodel (Bromocriptine Mesylate) This is an oral medication given to lower the level of prolactin. It may also be used to decrease the size of a pituitary tumor. This medication may be given to a woman wanting to become pregnant, because prolactin can interfere with the normal production of LH and FSH and therefore hinder ovulation.

Tests for prolactin are usually done in the morning, when raised levels are most noticeable. They should not be done following any

breast palpation, including during sexual activity, and/or following a breast examination done by the woman or her physician, as
this may result in a false positive result.

The dose of Parlodel is usually 1.25 to 3.75 mg taken daily at
bedtime. Side effects during the first few days may include dizziness,
nausea, headache, fatigue, and nasal congestion. These side effects
may be minimized if the dosage is increased gradually. Ovulation
may be expected within six weeks of starting Parlodel. However, it
is sometimes necessary for the specialist to prescribe Clomid simul-
taneously if you have not ovulated after two months on Parlodel.

Lupron (Leuprolide Acetate) This is a newer fertility drug that
has been used to treat endometriosis. For endometriosis, it is
given in a single intramuscular injection monthly for six months.
As of this writing, the drug has not been specifically approved for
the treatment of infertility, although some physicians are pre-
scribing it for infertile women. It is often used presurgically,
before treating endometriosis, and with in vitro fertilization.
Some women claim that side effects from this medication are
similar to symptoms experienced during menopause. These
include hot flashes, headaches, acne, vaginal dryness, bone pain,
reduction of breast size, emotional changes such as depression,
and decreased libido. Lupron is usually given for no more than a
total of six months due to the possibility of bone loss.

Metrodin (Urofollitropin) Metrodin is a potent gonadotropic substance used to stimulate follicle growth. It is given to women who
have polycystic ovaries, have elevated LH/FSH, or do not respond
to Clomid. After Metrodin is administered, it must be followed by
hCG. Women receiving Metrodin will be examined at least every
other day during the treatment and twice weekly after the treatment has ceased. Couples are reminded to have intercourse daily,
beginning on the day prior to treatment with hCG until ovulation
is apparent from progesterone levels. Approximately 83 percent
of women who conceive while taking Metrodin will have single
births, and 17 percent will have multiple births.

hCG (Human Chorionic Gonadotropin) When Humagon or
Metrodin have stimulated the growth of mature follicles, then

the woman will be given an injection of hCG to stimulate the release of the eggs from the follicles. It is usually recommended that the couple have intercourse daily, starting on the day prior to the hCG shot, up until ovulation occurs. Ovulation is confirmed by basal body temperature (BBT) charts, change in cervical mucus, and a positive pregnancy test. When the woman becomes pregnant she produces her own hCG, which stimulates the corpus luteum, a body formed in the ovary that produces progesterone. This is the main hormone of pregnancy and is the stimulus for many of the mother's physical changes during pregnancy. It is the hormone that home pregnancy tests detect.

Women who have been given hCG occasionally complain of tenderness at the injection site. Some hCG users experience minor side effects such as hot flashes, fluid retention, and headaches.

Luteal-Phase Problems

The luteal phase occurs during the second half of the menstrual cycle. After you ovulate, the part of the ovary that releases the egg becomes the corpus luteum, which produces progesterone, which prepares the uterus for egg implantation. When the luteal phase is shorter than normal, or if the amount of progesterone secreted is less than normal, the woman is considered to have a luteal-phase problem.

Women with luteal-phase problems often miscarry because the uterus is not ready for the egg's implantation. A blood test after ovulation usually detects the low blood progesterone associated with luteal-phase problems. Endometrial biopsies may also be done. Women who become pregnant with luteal-phase problems may have early spotting and, unless treated, may miscarry. Treatment includes progesterone, clomiphene, or hCG. Up to 15 percent of infertile women have luteal-phase problems.

Endometriosis

Endometriosis is another potential cause of infertility, affecting as many as 7 percent of women of childbearing age. It is often detected only after a woman reports that she is unable to conceive. Fragments of the endometrium, the uterine tissue, lodge in areas such as the abdominal cavity, ovaries, fallopian tubes, or bowel. Each month at the time of menses, these growths of tissue bleed in small amounts, stimulating the body to form scar tissue or adhesions.

Endometriosis may be mild, moderate, or severe. Some women with mild to moderate endometriosis have no symptoms, while others may experience very painful periods, painful intercourse, and abnormal bleeding. Pain alone, however, is not indicative of endometriosis, nor is it indicative of the severity of the problem.

The cause of endometriosis remains unclear. One theory is that during a woman's period, blood carrying tissue from inside the uterus is moved into the fallopian tubes. This tissue then adheres to other organs in the pelvis and peritoneum. Other researchers suspect certain immunological factors, such as the formation of antiendometrial antibodies or alterations in prostaglandin inhibitors. Women with a family history of endometriosis and women who have never had children are generally thought to be at a greater risk. Some researchers claim that most women experience some degree of endometriosis; but for unknown reasons, possibly an altered immune response, not every woman reacts to this condition in the same way.

There are also several theories as to how endometriosis affects fertility. These include ovulatory dysfunction, impaired tubal transport, hormonal and immunological factors, disturbed implantation of the egg, and subsequent spontaneous abortion.

A specialist who suspects endometriosis may recommend a laparoscopy to determine the extent of the problem. During the procedure, he or she may decide to remove the scar tissue. Afterward, oral contraceptives or progestin may be prescribed to suppress the body's natural hormonal secretions, thus reducing the chance of recurrence.

Treatments for endometriosis vary according to the severity of the problem. The newest medications used are gonadotropin-releasing hormone agonists. Pain is usually relieved within two to three months of treatment. Lupron injections can be given once a month for six months or Nafarelin nasal spray, prescribed at 200 mg twice a day for three to six months. Each of these medications can produce side effects, such as hot flashes, headaches, depression, and bone loss. Sometimes low-dose estrogen and progestin are added to reduce the negative effects. Danazol is a synthetic hormone that shrinks endometrial tissue. It is taken as a pill, pre-scribed at 200 to 400 mg, twice a day. Like Lupron, Danazol sup-presses female hormones, causing artificial menopause. Side effects may include weight gain, water retention, cessation of menses, decreased breast size, acne, oily skin, hot flashes, and mood swings.

Moderate to severe endometriosis may be treated with both surgery and medication. Some physicians use various types of lasers and advanced laparoscopic surgery. The first laser surgery was per-formed in 1974 by Dr. Joseph Bellina. Today, the technique has been refined and it is no longer a particularly long or delicate surgery. With the help of television cameras, lasers are used through a laparoscope to remove small adhesions in the fallopian tubes. Studies have indicated that pregnancy rates after surgery for women with moderate endometriosis can be as high as 47 percent, rates for those with severe endometriosis as high as 38 percent. However, studies have also shown decreased pregnancy rates when using in vitro fertilization (IVF) following laparoscopic surgery. IVF is often the best treatment option for infertile couples, so some women with mild endometriosis may choose to bypass this surgery in order to better their chances for a successful IVF pregnancy.

One woman shares her experience with endometriosis:

When I was in my early twenties, I was told I had endometriosis and that achieving pregnancy might pose a problem. We were married for a little more than two years when we decided to start a family. I thought that we'd better start trying because I was thirty-four and my husband was forty. Psychologically we prepared ourselves for long months of trying and infertility investigations. We didn't look forward to it all. Then came the big surprise ... about six weeks after we began trying to con-ceive, I got a positive pregnancy test. I was shocked and unpre-pared at the same time. I quickly adapted to the idea, but really one never knows how long it will take to become pregnant. You should be prepared the moment you start trying.

Pelvic Inflammatory Disease (PID)

Certain infections and illnesses may affect fertility. Infections in the pelvic area leave scar tissue behind, which interferes with conception. This condition, called pelvic inflammatory disease, is the cause of about 20 percent of all infertility problems in women, and this number is increasing. The National Institute of Allergy and Infectious Diseases estimates that about one million cases of PID occur annually, and more than one hundred thousand women become infertile each year as a result. The more sexual partners a woman has, the greater is her risk of developing PID. The disease is very difficult to diagnose because it either causes no symptoms or the symptoms it does produce—such as fever, abdominal pain, and vaginal bleeding—are also symptoms of various other disorders. PID may be associated with the use of the IUD and/or a history of sexually transmitted diseases.

Sexually Transmitted Diseases (STDs)

Genital herpes, genital warts, syphilis, gonorrhea, trichomonas, and chlamydia may lead to difficulties in becoming pregnant. A study done in 1985 at the Hutchinson Cancer Research Center in Seattle indicated that women with a history of gonorrhea had twice the chance of having problems conceiving due to fallopian-tube abnormalities, and that a history of trichomonas was also associated with fallopian-tube problems.

Among the one million women who contract STDs each year, as many as 150,000 to 200,000 will have infertility problems. Some classic symptoms of infection include low-grade fever, fatigue, dull pains in the pelvis, sharp sensations in the pelvis or bladder area, and painful intercourse. If you have any of these symptoms, you should see your gynecologist. Tell him or her about your symptoms; they might not be discernible during an examination. A sample should be taken of your vaginal discharge and/or growths and examined under a microscope. The sample will then be sent to a laboratory for a more detailed analysis. A medication may or may not be prescribed at that time.

Polycystic Ovaries (Stein-Leventhal Syndrome)

This is a condition brought on when ovulation has not occurred for an unusually long period of time, causing cysts to be formed on the ovaries. This problem is often associated with abnormal hormonal secretions and may produce symptoms such as irregular periods, excessive hair growth, and a tendency toward obesity.

The problem originates in the pituitary gland, the master gland that triggers the release of hormones in various parts of the body. Blood tests reveal this hormonal imbalance. About 75 percent of women with polycystic ovaries respond well to fertility medications. In some cases, laparoscopic surgery is carried out to remove the ovarian cysts.

One woman shares her experience:

> Because I had excessive hair growth even before I decided to start a family, one physician thought that I had this problem. He did many tests and investigations, all of which had normal results. Despite these results, when I was eighteen, he still told me I might have infertility problems one day. I laughed and said that excessive hair growth runs in my family. Ironically, he was right; I did have infertility problems, but for different reasons.

Cervical, Vaginal, and Anatomical Disorders

Disorders such as inadequate cervical mucus, cervical infections, or cauterization (the destruction of tissue with an electrical current, sometimes used to control bleeding after surgery) may affect fertility since mucus interacts in a specific way with sperm.

About the ninth or tenth day of the menstrual cycle, cervical mucus starts to increase and the cervix opens slightly to facilitate sperm entry. A common cause of infertility is the "cervical factor," meaning that the woman does not produce an adequate amount or quality (the wrong pH) of cervical mucus to facilitate easy sperm entry into the uterus. Some believe this is caused by a hormonal imbalance. Some physicians prescribe Robitussin cough syrup to loosen up the mucus. Others may recommend intrauterine insemination, in which a small catheter is introduced into the cervix leading into the uterus for implantation.

One woman describes the cause of her infertility problem:

> My vaginal mucosa was too acidic and I was producing an environment that killed my husband's sperm. [Normally the

vagina is acidic—the cervical fluid is alkaline, as is the spermatic fluid.] My physician recommended, after many long years of infertility investigations, that I douche with baking soda and water, an alkaline solution, prior to intercourse. I was pregnant with twin boys within four months.

Inadequate cervical mucus (i.e., inadequate in amount or consistency) may be treated by the use of estrogens such as Premarin. The dose of Premarin varies from .625 to 1.25 mg daily prior to ovulation. If after a few months you are still not pregnant, some specialists may recommend another form of treatment, such as cryosurgery. This is a painless procedure that involves freezing and has many applications, but in the case of infertility it serves to freeze the cervical area. It results in a sloughing off of the old cervical layers and the promotion of healing. It causes a temporary change in cervical mucosa, making it more profuse and watery.

Daughters of women who took DES during pregnancy may have anatomical abnormalities that may affect their fertility. Menstrual irregularities, cervical-mucus production problems, and anatomical abnormalities of the reproductive system, such as an abnormally shaped uterus, have in some cases been associated with DES usage. If you are a DES daughter, you must alert your physician. A careful gynecological examination will be done, including a Pap smear and special cervical tests.

Environmental Factors

Certain environmental factors may affect fertility and may also have the ability to cause miscarriage. For example, the rubber, leather, and dry-cleaning industries use the solvent benzene, which may affect fertility. Flight attendants exposed to high altitudes, hospital employees exposed to anesthesia, chemicals, and radiation, and those working irregular shifts and/or exposed to stress may also be adversely affected.

Advanced Age

The current social trend is for women to wait longer than previous generations did before starting their families. When they finally decide to have children, it may be some time before they become pregnant. This is because most women are at their reproductive peak between the ages of twenty and twenty-five. As we get older, our reproductive system undergoes physiological changes that may affect fertility. In general, there is a reduction in the number of eggs that are capable of forming a viable embryo. The follicles that do ovulate may be less hardy than they were when the woman was in her twenties. As a result, most women over the age of thirty-five have fewer viable eggs and may even ovulate less often. In addition, the incidence of endometriosis increases as women get older. Some clinicians suggest running a blood test on women over the age of thirty-five to check follicle-stimulating hormone (FSH) levels. Performed on the second or third day of a woman's cycle, this test determines whether or not her eggs are still fertile.

Nutrition and Exercise

What you eat may affect your ovulation and menstrual cycles. Studies have shown that diets low in protein may result in irregular menstrual cycles. Any extreme weight loss or weight gain can affect a woman's menstrual cycle and fertility.

Lack of body fat may result in irregular periods and infertility. The body's fat tissues store and convert hormones, including estrogen. To allow for the normal rise and fall of hormones, women must have a body fat content of about 22 percent.

Obesity may also affect fertility, because when a woman is obese she has a lot of fatty tissue, which produces extra estrogen. This works like a built-in birth control pill. It is common for obese women not to ovulate.

Regular and vigorous exercise may alter your menstrual cycle, according to the American College of Gynecologists and Obstetricians. Occasionally, menstrual periods may stop completely. This is especially true of long-distance runners. The college states that the degree of change in fertility brought about through regular exercise depends upon the individual woman. For example, some women may notice changes after doing twenty to thirty miles of running each week, while others may experience changes only after running as much as forty to sixty miles per week.

UNEXPLAINED INFERTILITY

The causes of infertility are not always known, and it is even difficult to document the incidence of unexplained infertility in the population. Researchers have noted that in 10 to 15 percent of couples who undergo investigation for infertility, the cause will not be identified, yet as many as 60 percent of these couples will eventually conceive without infertility treatment within three years. In some instances, the specialist may choose to repeat certain tests, such as sperm count, if all other test results prove normal. Other areas that are often investigated include sexual problems, such as timing and positions, and certain rare bacterial infections.

Treatment for unexplained infertility often presents a challenge for the health care team. Some specialists recommend a treatment of Clomid or Humagon, or both to stimulate egg-follicle production. This is usually followed by intercourse at the time of ovulation or, if that is not possible, artificial insemination with the partner's sperm. Often this is recommended before other invasive procedures such as in vitro fertilization (IVF), gamete intrafallopian transfer (GIFT), or ZIFT are performed.

EMOTIONAL FACTORS IN INFERTILITY

Infertility is very stressful for everyone involved. It is as difficult for the anxious grandparents as it is for the physician who wants to find the source of the infertility. And of course, it is especially stressful for the couple. It is common to develop feelings of hopelessness, as your specialist sends you for more and more tests and pregnancy seems to become only a dream. Sexual relations become a chore that must be performed at certain times of the month; the pure joy of sex is lost. For many infertile couples, tension only complicates the situation and makes conception that much more difficult. It is very much a catch-22 situation. One woman shares her thoughts:

> When I was trying to become pregnant, the days seemed like eternity as I waited for the signs of pregnancy. My childhood nightmares of childlessness became vivid, and as I faced the real possibility I grew to dislike myself more and more. The

key to my strength was a loving and supportive husband who always had an intuitive feeling that our lives would be blessed with children.

Obviously we cannot rule out the role that emotions play in our lives. It would not be far-fetched to assume that they also play some role (whether large or small) in our ability to conceive. Since there are few studies and there is no great body of knowledge about the subject, much of what is known is based on clinical assumptions rather than on hard facts backed up by research. Some studies, however, have indicated that the failure of women to menstruate during wartime may be one example of the effect that emotions have on fertility. Other studies have shown that wives of soldiers fail to menstruate when their husbands go to war.

Some earlier studies have noted that emotional tension may cause the fallopian tubes to go into spasms, thus hindering the egg's implantation. Other research indicates that chronic stress can reduce GnRH release from the hypothalamus, resulting in a reduction in FSH and LH. This reduction can result in anovulation (the suppression of ovulation).

As indicated earlier, sperm count may be affected by stress. Sperm production requires a lot of energy and is certainly subject to a temporary decrease by situations such as drug use, hot baths, stress, lack of sleep, or illness.

The issue of stress and fertility is a highly controversial and emotionally charged one. In general, we do not like being told that our mind controls our body. Yet, we are all no doubt familiar with stories of women who were unable to have children after years of trying, and who became pregnant shortly after choosing to adopt a child.

Women who have been trying to become pregnant may feel guilty. They may feel that something they did in the past is causing their present inability to become pregnant. Some may believe, irrationally, that it is some sort of punishment for previous wrongdoings. However, properly performed abortions, unusual sexual practices, and masturbating do not result in infertility. Any strong feelings of guilt or self-blame should be discussed with a trained counselor.

Some women with infertility problems develop a negative self-image, and as a result of this, their progress in their careers may be affected. This altered self-image may also lead a woman to resent her spouse and/or her colleagues. Some women become so totally absorbed in their infertility problems that everything they do and say revolves around their inability to have children. As one woman who had been trying to conceive for over two years told me,

> I was totally obsessed with trying to become pregnant. The thoughts were with me day in and day out. It encompassed everything and anything that I did. For more than two years I did not buy clothes for myself because I kept believing I would soon be pregnant and would need maternity clothes. I didn't expect to have so much difficulty, and instead of taking each day at a time I was really living in a fantasy world.

Dealing with Others

How you cope with your feelings about infertility will depend to a large extent on how those around you react to your problem. Somehow questions such as "So when are you going to start having children?" always seem to come up, whether at work or during social engagements. Comments such as "So, what are you waiting for?" or "You would make such wonderful parents" or "You don't have any children; don't you like children?" tend to magnify the pressure already felt by the infertile couple.

According to RESOLVE, a national support group for infertile couples, the inability to have children is considered a life crisis— one that can lead to a tremendous sense of isolation from friends and family, especially when there are other couples around with children. It is often a time of great loneliness. Feelings of anger and resentment are also very common among infertile couples. One woman shares her feelings about dealing with other people:

> I found it very difficult to talk with other people about my inability to conceive. It was particularly difficult at work, where everyone was my age and had one or more children. Seeing pictures on their desks and hearing them talk about

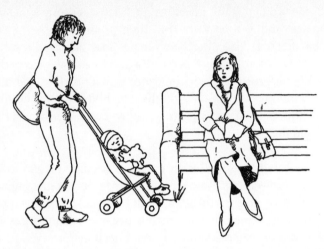

their kids was a constant reminder of my inadequacy. I also found it very difficult to share the joy of those women who were pregnant at work. I was both resentful and envious. I was invited to many baby showers but could not attend any because of these feelings. I just kept backing off from pregnant women.

Husbands play a crucial role in how women cope with infertility. Many women say that having a supportive and understanding husband made a tremendous difference to them during this time. The stresses of infertility can also strongly tax the marital relationship. Lovemaking becomes only a means of becoming pregnant, and spontaneity becomes a thing of the past. One woman admits,

At one point I thought what was once a strong marriage would end. You were told when and how to have sex, and you would end up accusing your husband of not trying when he should have been trying. To tell a man when he has to perform is very difficult. There was an enormous amount of emotional strain. To survive an infertility problem you must have a very, very strong marriage.

Others say that other family members may be either helpful or harmful:

Sometimes dealing with family members is not so easy. I remember I had this aunt with five kids who had seven pregnancies in six years with two miscarriages. She said, "Oh, why are you doing all this [taking Humagon, temperature charts, etc.], you are crazy! If you can't have kids, you can't have kids. If God wanted you to have kids, you'd have kids."

Another woman says,

It got to a point that whenever I saw pregnant women on the street I really envied them. It got so intense sometimes that when I saw a mother being rotten to her child I would speak up and say, "Listen, you're really lucky you have that child at all."

Often women find, through talking with others, that there are many infertile couples. Speaking with others and joining support groups such as Resolve, Inc., help dispel the feeling that you are all alone with your problem.

Infertility Counseling

Some couples benefit from professional counseling if the problem of infertility is creating undue stress in their lives or if they are uncomfortable in the milieu of support groups. Generally, you will be asked to attend sessions as a couple. Although only one partner may have an infertility problem, this approach underscores the fact that it is a problem that must be resolved jointly, under medical supervision. Your counselor will assess the degree of stress that infertility has placed on your relationships. The counselor will also explore the methods you use to cope with stress, the kind of expectations you have for the medical interventions, and your plans if pregnancy is impossible.

It is helpful to have someone who will listen to your concerns. In many instances, partners may say things in the presence of a counselor that they might not otherwise disclose to each other. This often sheds light on crucial issues for both partners. Counseling may also help you work through disappointment and loss and may lead to a more realistic and productive approach to problems of infertility.

Chapter 2

———————— O ————————

Infertility Testing

Today, there is hope for infertile couples. Medical technology is finding new solutions, and women who not so long ago may have had to settle for remaining childless are having children.

Sometimes, the chances of conceiving successfully are increased by making simple changes in the way you and your partner make love. Here are some ideas:

Conception Tips

O Have intercourse every day during your fertile time.

O Have your hips elevated on a pillow with knees bent during intercourse.

O Refrain from using lubricants.

O Have your partner remain inside your vagina for a short time following ejaculation.

O Stay in bed for at least thirty minutes following intercourse.

O Don't douche for at least one hour after intercourse.

If you have been trying for more than a year to get pregnant and you have used some of the conception tips listed above, then you should review your situation with your physician. If you have a general practitioner or an obstetrician-gynecologist, he or she may begin some preliminary testing before referring you to an infertility specialist. Some of these tests include a pelvic exam, a check of basal body temperature (BBT) charts, and monitoring some baseline hormone levels, such as prolactin and progesterone, during certain parts of the menstrual cycle. Some physicians may also recommend a postcoital test or diagnostic laparoscopy. (These tests are discussed in greater detail later.) Depending upon the results, he or she may refer you to a specialist.

CHOOSING A SPECIALIST

Some women find it difficult starting a new relationship with another physician, especially in regard to a very sensitive subject like infertility. However, it is very important that you seek a specialist in order to obtain maximal results from your infertility investigations. You will get to know your physician well during the course of the next few months, and it is important that you choose one whom you feel comfortable with and who is competent.

Below are some questions you may want to ask during your first appointment.

○ How long have you been in practice?

○ What percentage of your patients have infertility problems?

○ What percentage of your patients have been successfully treated for infertility?

○ How do you plan to approach my case?

○ Which tests are done first?

○ Are the tests done concurrently or consecutively?

○ Are both partners investigated at the same time?

○ How long will the infertility investigation take?

○ Do you have days for seeing infertile couples, or must I sit in a waiting room full of pregnant women?

○ If I call your office with a question, do I speak with you or an assistant?

○ What are your office hours?

○ What happens if I have a question on the weekend or if I ovulate on the weekend or on a holiday?

○ What are the fees for the services you offer?

○ How do you handle medical insurance?

It is important that your partner be present at the first and, in many cases, all the appointments. The first thing your specialist will determine is whether you actually have a fertility problem. He or she will do a complete medical history and physical examination. You will be asked many questions, such as when you began menstruating, the nature of your menstrual cycle (i.e., flow, duration), previous pregnancies, the nature of your sexual relations, and any health problems or diseases you have had in the past. You may be asked about your social and professional life and whether you are taking any medications. Some questions, such as those about your sexual relationships, may make you feel uncomfortable; however, you should remember that these questions are being asked so that the specialist can form a clear picture in order to help you. Try to provide as many details as possible.

During your first meeting you should determine if the specialist speaks to you in a logical and unhurried fashion so that you can understand everything he or she is talking about. You should feel a good connection during this first visit, and you should leave the appointment feeling positive. After this first visit you should have some idea of your specialist's medical strategy for you and your partner. If there is a "wait and see" approach, it may be a good idea to change specialists, since you have probably already waited for a year or more without results.

If you are dissatisfied with the specialist and want to make a change, it is important to notify him or her of the reason for your decision. In general, honesty is the best policy. Often, changing is not as important as seeking a second opinion, especially when surgery has been recommended. Most professionals understand the need for second opinions. Peer review is one of the most efficient ways of weeding out the qualified from the unqualified. You should also remember that differing opinions do not always mean that one person is right and the other is wrong. There may be different solutions to a problem. We tend to gravitate toward those whose solutions we agree with. If you go for a second opinion, remember to bring your medical records and test results.

FEMALE INVESTIGATIONS

Basal Body Temperature (BBT)

This is the temperature that you take first thing in the morning before getting up. It provides the information that helps determine if you are ovulating. A special thermometer may be purchased with an expanded and easy-to-read scale. These thermometers usually come with graph paper, or your specialist will provide a chart.

Progesterone is the hormone responsible for an increase in your temperature, and it is released into your bloodstream only after you ovulate. In about 25 to 50 percent of women with normal ovulation, their BBT decreases slightly at ovulation and then rises as progesterone levels increase. The rise may be indicated as a jump of about 6/10 of a degree (six lines on your graph).

Keep your thermometer, graph paper, and a pencil at your bedside. Take your temperature before rising, drinking, smoking, or walking. It is very important not to miss a day. Make this as routine as brushing your teeth.

After a few months of following your charts, your specialist will be able to detect a pattern. You may be ovulating each month, not ovulating at all, or ovulating sporadically every other month or so.

Some studies have shown that BBT charts can be inaccurate predictors of ovulation for some women. If this is true for you, home-testing kits are an ideal option.

LH Dipstick

New home-testing kits have become available to detect ovulation before it occurs, without taking your temperature. These kits predict the day of ovulation based on urine samples. Some of these include Answer Ovulation Test, Clearplan Easy Ovulation Predictor, OvuKIT Self-Test, OvuQuick Self-Test, and First Response Ovulation Predictor Test. These urine tests measure the hormone LH in your urine, which reaches a high level in your bloodstream and urine about twenty-four hours prior to ovulation. If you do the urine dipstick each morning, the test will be

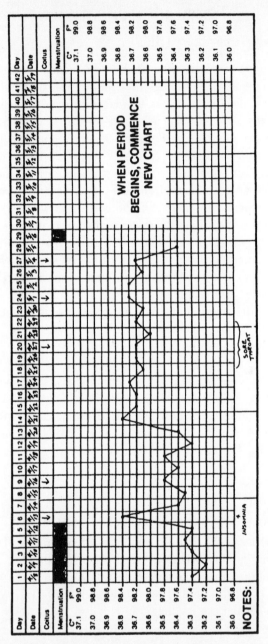

Basal Body Temperature Chart
(Courtesy of Merrell Dow Pharmaceuticals, Inc.)

negative until the day of your LH surge. If you do the test a day or two later, it will be negative. Ovulation should occur thirty-six to forty-eight hours after the LH starts to increase and about twenty-four hours after it reaches its peak. This method helps you pinpoint the day before ovulation, which will help you determine when you ovulate.

Before purchasing a kit, it is a good idea to find out when the urine sample should be collected. Some tests require a midday collection, which could be inconvenient for working women.

Tips on Using Ovulation Predictors at Home

○ Have all materials ready before beginning the test.

○ Follow the directions on the label exactly as they are written.

○ Do the test at the same time each day in the same room with the same lighting.

○ Do not drink large quantities of water prior to the test (water dilutes urine and affects test results).

○ Tell your physician about any medications you are taking (test results may be altered by certain medications).

○ Do not use any contraceptives.

○ Look for the first noticeable change in color, not the darkest.

○ Remember that not all women ovulate each month.

○ If you have any questions, ask your pharmacist or physician, or call the toll-free number included with your testing kit.

Endometrial Biopsy

This is a biopsy of a few cells scraped from the endometrium or inner lining of the uterus. The test is usually done to detect whether there is adequate progesterone to prepare the uterus for egg implantation. If the uterus does not develop properly, this is usually due to inadequate amounts of progesterone. The biopsy is done after ovulation, which is detected with the BBT charts, and usually a few days prior to the start of the next menstrual period.

It is usually done in your physician's office. You will experience a slight amount of pain or cramping. It is normal to have slight spotting for a few days after the procedure.

The procedure involves inserting a plastic catheter or pipette through the cervix into the uterus to obtain a piece of uterine lining for analysis. In some cases a lowered progesterone level is not apparent in blood tests but may be identified through an endometrial biopsy.

Postcoital or Hühner Test

From the BBT charts your physician will ascertain when you ovulate. The next time you ovulate (plus or minus a few days), you may be asked to return to the office for a postcoital or Hühner test. Recent studies show that this procedure is not a good predictor of fertility; however, some clinics continue to find it useful.

The postcoital test is designed to see if your cervix is producing fertile mucus. This mucus enables sperm to live and travel in your reproductive system. After abstaining for forty-eight hours, you and your partner will be asked to have intercourse within six hours before your appointment. Your specialist will then take a sample of the mucus from your cervix. This sample will be closely examined in the laboratory.

If your cervical environment is not compatible with sperm motility, it may mean you are too early in the cycle. The test may then be repeated in forty-eight hours if you have not yet ovulated. A semen analysis will also be done to determine the quality and number of your partner's sperm.

Some practitioners believe that the results of this test may be inaccurate or falsely negative. The rationale is that there are only a few days each month when the woman's cervical mucus is of the correct consistency to allow sperm penetration. Therefore, if this test were done at the wrong time of the month, it would be difficult to ascertain if this test was evaluating the cervical mucus or the fertility of the sperm.

One woman describes her test results:

We were trying to have a baby for nearly three years before we sought help. Finally we were investigated, and among the

tests was the Hühner test, which placed all my difficulties in
a nutshell. The test showed that my husband's sperm were
not surviving in my cervical mucus. They were dying off
immediately upon contact. I was advised to douche with bak-
ing soda and water prior to intercourse, and lo and behold! I
became pregnant within three months. Sometimes there are
simple solutions to what seem to be complex problems.

Ultrasound

The development of a transvaginal ultrasound helps specialists to
safely examine the developing ovarian follicles and to see the dis-
integration of the follicle, which is an indication that ovulation
has occurred. This exam can cost as much as $800, compared to
$30 for a dipstick kit. However, it is the most precise way of
determining when ovulation has occurred. It is done in a matter
of minutes and is now used to monitor women who are taking
ovulation-stimulating medications.

Unlike the abdominal ultrasound, this procedure is best done
on an empty bladder. The procedure is done by placing a rubber
glove or condom over the ultrasound transducer with a special
lubricant on the tip. This is then placed into the vagina and the
technician or specialist sees the ovaries and uterus on a TV
screen. This test may reveal very small uterine fibroids and determine how thick the uterine lining is and how well the uterus is
responding to hormone production. If the lining is thin, this indicates that there is low hormone production.

This test is a safe alternative to laparoscopy and is usually no
more uncomfortable than a pelvic exam. For more information,
see chapter 7.

Hysterosalpingogram (HSG)

The HSG is an X-ray of the internal reproductive system done if
the specialist suspects that tubal, uterine, or abdominal problems
may be causing your infertility. This X-ray enables the specialist
to identify any abnormalities, such as blockages, adhesions, or
anatomical problems. It is usually done in the hospital's radiology
department two to six days after the end of your menstrual period

but prior to ovulation. If you are scheduled for this test but have vaginal bleeding or any type of infection in your reproductive system, you should notify your physician. The test will probably be postponed until these symptoms subside.

The procedure involves injecting a radio-opaque or iodine-based dye through the cervix and then taking a series of X-ray pictures. If your tubes are open without obstruction, this liquid should go freely through the cervix and into the uterus and fallopian tubes. Your physician will be able to see this passage on a TV screen beside you. Some women say that the test feels like they are having intense menstrual cramps. For most women, the test is uncomfortable, but the discomfort does not last long. In some instances, women complain of feeling weak and queasy afterward. Most providers offer antibiotics to help prevent the risk of infection. This is not a surgical procedure and does not require hospitalization.

The HSG has replaced tubal insufflation (Rubin's test) because it provides more information about the female reproductive system. Some studies have shown increased conception rates as early as three to six months after the test.

Laparoscopy

The HSG does not always show scarring on the outside of the fallopian tubes; to detect this a laparoscopy may be necessary. Laparoscopy used to be a fairly common test in the infertility investigation. It involves passing a surgical telescope—a long metal tube with a lens at one end and a fiber-optic light source at the other end—into the abdomen through a small incision made near the navel. It is done under general anesthesia and therefore a day in the hospital is usually necessary.

The laparoscope allows the specialist to identify and evaluate the abdominal cavity and its organs, including the uterus and ovaries. Laparoscopy is the only firm way to diagnose endometriosis. Although this procedure is usually done prior to planned surgery for endometriosis, skilled physicians may repair mild adhesions on the fallopian tubes through the telescope device. This is done by cutting through adhesions using operating instruments attached to the end of the telescope or inserted through a second incision.

Many couples planning to use in vitro fertilization skip this step. Women with mild endometriosis can go straight into IVF procedures without a laparoscopy.

Hysteroscopy

A hysteroscopy is another type of investigation involving an internal examination of the uterus, requiring the insertion of a tube through the cervix into the uterus. The tube has a special fiber-optic light to assist the physician in detecting any abnormalities of the uterus, such as lesions or tumors. It may be done in your physician's office or in the outpatient department of the hospital using local anesthesia. It is often done at the same time as a laparoscopy.

Additional Tests

Other diagnostic investigations may include hormone, urine, and blood tests to determine whether you have too much or too little of any one hormone and to identify any abnormal structures in the reproductive system, such as tumors or fibroids. The length of time it takes to explore the reasons for infertility varies.

MALE INVESTIGATIONS

Most specialists working with a couple will evaluate the male partner's fertility regardless of the female partner's test results, in order to obtain a full picture of the couple's fertility. The tests done on men are initially much simpler than those for women.

During the first appointment, the physician will take a medical history and try to identify certain risk factors such as a history of mumps, an undescended testicle, genital infections, urologic surgery, and any exposure to environmental toxins. In addition, they may perform certain basic tests.

Urine Analysis

A complete urine analysis is done to detect certain disorders. A urinalysis can identify any bacteria or white blood cells, which may indicate an infection in the urinary system or in the prostate gland. A concentration of sperm in the urine is indicative of retrograde ejaculation (sperm going back into the bladder instead of forward into the penis).

Hormone Tests

Blood tests will be performed in order to give the specialist a baseline of the male's hormonal status. Testosterone, the primary male hormone, will be assessed, as it is associated with sex drive and erection. FSH and LH levels will be determined, as these are involved in the testicular functions.

Sperm Count

Sperm count is the number of sperm in the ejaculate. The term is sometimes used to mean the total number of sperm (the total sperm count) and at other times the number of sperm per milliliter (the sperm concentration).

To obtain a sperm count the couple is advised to abstain for a few days, and then the male is asked to produce a semen specimen by masturbation, deposit it into a clear glass jar, and deliver it to the laboratory within one hour of ejaculating. Some men may find it difficult to masturbate and may be given a special plastic condom to be used to collect the sperm during sexual intercourse. It is preferable, however, to use the former method, as some practitioners claim that the materials out of which condoms are made, and sometimes the chemicals used to line the inside of the condoms, may damage or kill the sperm and so affect the sperm count.

The concentration of sperm is counted under a microscope, and the total sperm count is calculated and recorded. Regardless of the male's care in collecting the specimen and the laboratory's accuracy in performing the tests, there are frequent variations. Sperm counts should be repeated at least three times over the next few months. Certain conditions may also temporarily lower a man's sperm count. These include any infection, such as the flu, or undue stress.

Some men may show a zero sperm count. Those who have a zero sperm count should be tested for fructose, a sugar that the epididymis adds to the seminal fluid. If fructose is absent, this suggests a blockage in the reproductive tract that prevents the sperm from getting into the ejaculate. If fructose is present and there is a zero sperm count, this suggests a problem in the testicles' ability to manufacture sperm.

Sperm count alone may be a misleading indicator of a man's fertility. Sperm quantity does not necessarily mean that there is sperm quality. There may be many sperm incapable of penetrating the egg. There are other parameters, such as motility, that affect the sperm's ability to penetrate the egg. These parameters are examined during the semen analysis.

Semen Analysis

A semen analysis is a laboratory examination of the semen to check the quality and the quantity of the sperm. The specimen is collected in the same way as for a sperm count. Most specialists will recommend abstinence for three days. Because sperm counts and quality vary, at least three analyses are usually done.

The total volume of a normal ejaculation is between one-half and one teaspoon. However, the actual volume of ejaculate does not indicate the amount of sperm that is produced. Some men have very low ejaculate volumes, but they can have a high concentration of sperm in that volume. Typically, human male ejaculate contains sixty million or more sperm per cubic centimeter, and sperm that has good motility can propel itself up the woman's reproductive tract at a rate of about two inches an hour.

Semen analysis results will indicate the appearance of the semen, the time it takes to liquefy, and the actual volume. A low volume may indicate that the semen does not contain enough of the normal components of the ejaculate. For example, the seminal vesicles produce about 60 to 65 percent of the ejaculate, which includes the proteins causing the ejaculate to coagulate; and the prostate gland produces about 30 percent of the ejaculate, which contains enzymes that cause the ejaculate to liquefy.

As a consequence, if the semen does not look like clotted gel, then this suggests that the seminal vesicles are not making enough fluid or that these ducts may be blocked. On the other hand, if the semen looks clumpy, then this may indicate a prostate disorder or a relatively high frequency of intercourse.

A low volume of ejaculate may also indicate a low testosterone level. Testosterone is a male hormone responsible for stimulating the seminal vesicles to produce enough fluid. An unusually high semen volume may indicate an infection.

Some men may not have any ejaculate. This may be due to retrograde ejaculation, which causes the sperm to go backward into the bladder. This is usually related to diabetes, previous surgery, or certain blood pressure medications.

Computerized Analysis of Sperm Motion

The computer-assisted analysis of sperm motion assists the specialist in correlating sperm motility with fertility. Using the computer helps determine the sperm's swimming speed and how straight they swim. This is an automated method of grading the movement of the sperm. The sperm are rated on a scale of one to four. Grade-one sperm, which tend to wiggle in place with no forward progression, are unlikely to fertilize. Grade-four sperm tend to move in a very straight line very quickly and are therefore very likely to fertilize.

This analysis is done with the assistance of a video camera connected to a microscope. The input is transferred to a TV screen and then to a computer programmed to analyze sperm motion. The computer can automatically calculate the speed of the sperm in getting from point A to point B. The specialist then receives a printout of the report.

The Hamster Test

The Hamster Test is a test of the ability of a man's sperm to penetrate a hamster's egg stripped of its outer membrane, the zona pellucida. Basically, this is a trial test of in vitro fertilization, using a hamster's egg instead of the woman's. The test is very expensive and has undergone various modifications over the years.

Using enzymes, the lab technician removes the coating around the hamster egg (zona pellucida). This coating prevents interspecies fertilization and is also found on the human egg.

After the coating is removed, the male's sperm is mixed with the hamster eggs. The eggs are then collected to see how many have been penetrated by the sperm.

This test is used when the male has had a normal semen analysis and the woman has no identifiable fertility problem. It also is a trial to see if in vitro fertilization will work for the couple. This test has about a 90 percent accuracy rate. Like the sperm count test, it may have to be repeated in order to give the most accurate results.

Sperm Antibodies

Sometimes a man's body sees his sperm as invaders and produces antibodies against them. These antisperm antibodies attach themselves to the sperm's surface and may alter the sperm's ability to fertilize. Depending upon where they attach themselves, they may affect either the sperm's movement or the fertilization process itself.

Sperm antibodies are measured in the man's semen or in the blood. There are many theories as to why sperm antibodies occur in the male. For the most part, men produce antibodies against sperm only when the sperm comes into contact with their blood. When men are born, they have no sperm, and therefore when sperm develop, they are recognized by the body as "foreign." When sperm get into tissues, such as after reproductive surgery (e.g., a vasectomy) or injury, the body recognizes them as foreign and produces antibodies against them. An antisperm antibody test may be done if the man's sperm clumps, yet the man has no sign of infection. These are blood or seminal fluid tests.

A woman may also be allergic to her partner's sperm and consequently develop antibodies against the sperm. Treatment for sperm antibodies may include using condoms during intercourse for six months to reduce the woman's exposure to the sperm and/or taking low doses of the steroid dexamethasone for three months. If there are antibodies in the woman's cervical mucus, then both husband and wife will be given steroids. Sometimes the woman's mucus is "hostile" to the man's sperm and the woman may be treated with hormones to change the composition of her mucus. Some specialists may also recommend douching with either vinegar (which makes secretions more acidic) or bak-ing soda (which makes secretions more alkaline) to change the pH or acidity factor of the mucus.

Testicular Biopsy or Testicular Sperm Extraction (TESE)

This involves a microscopic inspection by a pathologist of a very small piece of testicular tissue. It may be recommended for the male who is not producing sperm, especially if his physical exam-ination is perfectly normal.

The procedure is done by removing a small sample of tissue from each testicle. It allows the pathologist to identify sperm in various stages of development. This is done on an outpatient basis, and usually no stitches are required. The man may return to work in one or two days and the results will be ready before the end of the week.

Vasography

A vasography is an X-ray study of the vas deferens. If the testic-ular biopsy shows there is normal sperm production, but there is no sperm in the ejaculate, this can indicate a blockage some-where in the reproductive system. In this case, the specialist will perform a vasography to identify the location of the blockage. It is important to note that this test is usually not necessary to diag-nose an obstruction, but it may be used as part of an operation to fix the obstruction.

A vasogram is performed by making a small incision in the scrotum and exposing the vas deferens. A special dye is injected into the vas deferens and X-rays are taken from various angles.

O

Over the last decade, the number of infertile couples has slowly begun to drop. At the same time, the number of couples seeking infertility treatments has increased dramatically. According to the Centers for Disease Control, more than 65,800 pregnancy attempts were made in 1996 using assisted reproductive technol-ogy. This figure represents an 11 percent increase from 1995. This increase may be the result of several factors. Some claim that as the demographics of our population change, so do the trends. The baby boom generation, no longer in their prime reproductive years, may be looking to infertility treatments as a way to continue having children. Some researchers claim that most women today marry later, develop a career, and then try to become pregnant. By the time modern couples decide to have children, usually in their thirties, they are just not as fertile as they were when they were younger. Revolutionary advances in infertility treatments have made late-life pregnancy an option. Information, advanced procedures, and medications are more accessible today than ever before.

Even so, infertility maintains a certain stigma. The most well-meaning people may have a difficult time accepting it. Evidence of this is the frequently made remark "Oh, you just need a holiday," an unthinking attempt to explain away a couple's infertility.

Some women, pressured by society's expectations and their own intense desire to have a child, are driven to desperation, as this rather humorous poem shows:

> Anything. Anything. I'll do anything.
> Temperature charts, Test-Tape, litmus paper. Abstinence to maximize sperm count.
> Lying on my back with a pillow under my behind and my legs up like a beetle.
> Vitamin A. Vitamin E. Zinc, Manganese.
> Anything. I'll do anything—but please—oh please—don't ask me to just relax.

HELPFUL PUBLICATIONS

Wanting a Child by Jill Bialosky and Helen Schulman (editors)

Chapter 3

———————— O ————————

Positive Alternatives
for the Infertile Couple

Despite all the investigations and possible treatments, some couples are still unable to conceive. This does not mean, however, that they will live a life of childlessness. In light of advancing medical technology, there is more hope and there are more options for these couples. About 500,000 of the 2.7 million Americans with infertility problems can be helped through alternative methods. What follows are some alternatives used today. Some are very new and may be available only in highly specialized hospitals.

ADOPTION

Adoption is one of the oldest solutions for the infertile couple. However, because of the declining birthrate in Western society, adopting a child is not as easy now as it once was. The waiting lists are growing longer, and the available children are fewer and fewer in number. It is most difficult to adopt Caucasian babies; some states have a five-to-seven-year waiting period. Many couples are now open to considering adopting children of a different nationality or those with special needs. If you are willing to accept a child from a race other than your own or from another country, the waiting time may be shorter.

Most adoptions occur through social agencies, although there are still many "family adoptions" (within the person's own family) and private adoptions in which a physician or a lawyer makes the arrangements. Underground adoptions are also an option. However, they are quite expensive—ranging as high as $10,000 per adoption—and some people have serious doubts about the ethics of what has been called "baby farming." International adoptions, on average, cost around $20,000. This has become more popular over the last decade; however, hundreds of children are thought to be smuggled into the United States just for this purpose.

Recently, the Internet has become a hopeful tool, making it easier for families to find information on children needing new homes. In the United States, about one hundred thousand children—many with physical, mental, or emotional problems—are in foster homes. Online support groups and adoption resources may offer children without families a greater chance at finding a new home.

Adopting a child should be a positive experience. You should feel good about your decision. It is often very helpful to speak with others who have adopted, or to join a support group with other adoptive parents, such as those listed in Appendix C.

Some women who adopt experience a feeling of elation once their decision is made. They claim that they feel "pregnant" as they become excited and curious about their new child. Having the support of family and friends also helps in adapting to this new change in your life.

Over the years, adoption raises some controversial issues. As the children grow up they may want to meet their biological parents and understand their origins. Many believe that it is a human right to know one's biological parents. There are associations that help adoptees find their parents. Others, most often the adoptive parents, believe that searching for the biological parents is not a good idea.

ARTIFICIAL INSEMINATION

Artificial insemination (AI) is used primarily if there is an insoluble problem of male infertility whereby the sperm is borderline fertile, and if there has been little or no success after various attempts to increase the sperm count. It may also be recommended in certain cases of unexplained infertility or if the cervical mucus is hostile to sperm. Two methods of AI exist today: one using the woman's partner (artificial insemination husband—AIH) and the other using an anonymous donor (artificial insemination donor—AID). The sperm may be either fresh or frozen. Both methods are performed in the specialist's office.

Prior to the artificial insemination, the specialist will want to meet with both the man and woman. A consent form will have to be signed by both parties, stating that any children produced by AI will be their own legitimate children and their heirs, that they waive forever any right to disclaim such a child as their own, and that the nature of the agreement will make the use of AI confidential among the man, the woman, and the physician. The physician is also not to be held responsible for any fetal abnormalities.

Artificial insemination is carefully timed to coincide with ovulation, which is determined by basal body temperature charts, cervical mucus production, dilation and closure of the cervix, ultrasound, or LH dipstick. Sometimes the specialist prescribes Clomid, Humagon, or hCG to induce ovulation at a more predictable time and to minimize the stress of AI. Women who take medications to stimulate ovulation usually ovulate on the fourteenth day of their cycle. Studies have shown that the success of AI is increased if the woman's ovulation is artificially stimulated. If the woman is given ovulation stimulants (Menotropins), then ultrasound and estrogen testing is done to ensure the success of the medications.

If the choice is AIH, the procedure calls for the partner to ejaculate into a clean container. The woman is then inseminated the day after the hCG is given (usually the day before ovulation). The sperm are first prepared by a washing and are then deposited in the woman's vagina and cervix. Some physicians prefer to deposit the sperm directly into the uterus to increase the chances of fertilization. Both types of insemination are painless and take less than a minute to perform. An ultrasound is done afterward to see if a follicle appears. If it does not appear, the woman is inseminated again two days later.

The other method, AID, is recommended if the woman's partner is not producing sperm, if a woman prefers to be a single mother, or for lesbian couples wishing to have children. AID may also be done if a male does not want to pass on a genetic defect such as Downs syndrome, Tay-Sachs disease, or Huntington's Chorea, or if the couple has Rh problems or incompatibilities.

The procedure is the same as that for AIH. Most donors in the United States are medical students or residents. One of the best sperm banks in the United States is the California Cryobank, Inc., located in Westwood with labs across the country. They ship sperm all over the world and give a detailed pedigree of the donors, including physical characteristics, race, religion, nationality, education, and interests. (You can contact them by calling 800-231-3373 or visiting their website, www.cryobank.com.)

The donated sperm are carefully screened, and many centers today try to match the donor, the recipient, and the recipient's partner. The semen is also examined to ensure a sperm count of over 80 million/ml with good motility. Although there are screening procedures today to detect chromosomal and genetic abnormalities, it is a good idea to ask about the chromosomal analysis and genetic history of the donor's family. Screening tests for AIDS (Acquired Immune Deficiency Syndrome), sexually transmitted diseases, and other diseases are also done routinely. Because of the possible six-month incubation period of the AIDS virus, frozen sperm is usually used today because the donor can be observed for six months and will have a repeat blood test at that time. The success rate with AI is good: approximately 40 to 50 percent of all women who undergo this procedure will conceive within the first six cycles.

IN VITRO FERTILIZATION

In vitro fertilization (IVF), or the creation of "test-tube babies," is usually recommended when a woman has damaged or blocked fallopian tubes or severe pelvic adhesions. The technique may also be used for those with endometriosis, a partner with male infertility, or sperm-mucus problems, or in the event of unexplained infertility. Prior to in vitro fertilization, hormones such as Clomid, Humagon, Metrodin, or Lupron are given to stimulate egg production. Couples who choose in vitro fertilization undergo a thorough screening process and must meet certain criteria. The woman must have one normal ovary and no internal infections.

The woman's ovulation cycle is closely monitored through blood tests, ultrasound, and other examinations. Just before ovulation would naturally occur, transvaginal ultrasound is used to locate and retrieve the eggs. This procedure is usually done under light anesthesia; the woman will wake up quickly and probably go home in one or two hours. Today, with the help of medications such as Lupron and Humagon, specialists are able to obtain five times the number of eggs as in previous years. Nearly twenty to forty eggs are retrieved.

After laboratory examination to see if the egg is suitable for fertilization, it is placed in a culture media, somewhat similar to the environment of the fallopian tube, and put into an incubator.

The partner should provide his sperm about three hours before the procedure. This gives time for the sperm to be washed. (See the section on sperm washing below.)

The egg is mixed with newly ejaculated sperm, and with any luck fertilization will occur. (It is important for the man to abstain for forty-eight hours prior to giving the sperm specimen.) The covered dish is then placed in an incubator at normal body temperature and is examined from time to time under a microscope. Approximately forty-eight to seventy-two hours later, or when four to eight cells have been identified, the embryo is transferred through the woman's vagina into her uterus. The procedure is done in the physician's office with the woman lying on her back with knees up, as in a cervical exam. Sometimes the table is tilted about twenty degrees head-down. The vagina and cervix are cleaned, and then the solution from the test tube (the width of a thin straw) is inserted into the uterus through the vagina. The procedure takes a few moments and is done without anesthesia.

While the embryo is in the test tube, the woman will be prescribed progesterone in order to prepare her uterus for implantation and to increase the chances of success of the procedure. Some specialists recommend taking progesterone for the first few weeks of pregnancy to further increase the likelihood of success.

The first IVF baby—Louise Brown—was born in 1978 in England under the supervision of Dr. Robert Edwards and Dr. Patrick Steptoe. In June 1990, an issue of *Time* magazine claimed that this technique had produced approximately twenty thousand offspring. IVF may be both mentally, physically, and financially exhausting for the couple because of the high cost, the stress of the procedure, and the ongoing tests to determine the right time to perform the procedure. The technique costs anywhere from $6,000 to $10,000 per attempt. The procedure's results may be slow in coming, and the couple needs to have both patience and devotion. Success rates vary according to the mother's age and the number of embryos transferred. The implantation rate per embryo is about 15 to 20 percent; however, for women between the ages of twenty-three and twenty-nine the live-birth rate is as high as 43 percent per cycle.

Ultrasound-guided egg retrieval is one step beyond in vitro fertilization in that a woman does not have to have general anesthesia during the procedure. Instead, eggs are obtained through a needle passed through either the abdomen, the urethra, or the vaginal wall leading to the ovary. Because this procedure is performed with mild sedation or local anesthesia, and no incision is made, it is very attractive to those choosing in vitro fertilization as an alternative.

INTRACYTOPLASMIC SPERM INJECTION (ICSI)

Couples experiencing infertility as a result of low sperm count, antisperm antibodies, or a vasectomy will often benefit from intracytoplasmic sperm injection. Often, for one reason or another, the man's sperm are unable to penetrate the woman's egg. This relatively new procedure involves selecting a single sperm to be injected through a tiny needle directly into an egg. The resulting embryo is placed back into the woman's uterus, in the same manner as IVF. ICSI is used in conjunction with the other ART (assisted reproductive technologies) procedures mentioned here.

GAMETE INTRAFALLOPIAN TRANSFER (GIFT)

Gamete intrafallopian transfer is an alternative for couples who are unable to achieve pregnancy through other methods of fertility treatment. This alternative is useful for those with a long history of untreatable or unexplained infertility, severe male infertility, endometriosis, cervical problems, or immunological problems. However, to qualify for GIFT, a woman must have at least one open (patent) fallopian tube. The technique was developed in 1984 by Dr. Richardo H. Asch.

GIFT involves placing the eggs and the sperm, using a laparoscope, into the woman's fallopian tube so that fertilization may take place where it occurs naturally. Following fertilization in the fallopian tube, the egg makes its way to the uterus for implantation. Prior to undergoing this technique, the woman's body is prepared with hormones to stimulate the development of ovarian follicles so that there is a greater chance of retrieving several ripe eggs capable of being fertilized by the sperm. The hormonal injections include Humagon and/or Lupron, Metrodin, or Clomid, usually given from day three or four of the start of the last menstrual period for about seven to ten days. These medications are given until an ultrasound shows that the ovarian follicle measures about 5/8 inch (16 mm) in diameter. At this time the woman is admitted to the hospital for the GIFT procedure. The man is told to abstain from ejaculation for forty-eight hours prior to the procedure.

About two hours before this procedure, a semen sample is collected from the man and prepared for implantation. Through a laparoscope, the eggs are withdrawn from the ovarian follicle and then placed along with the sperm into a tube or catheter. The contents are then transferred to the fallopian tube. The procedure takes forty to sixty minutes.

The success rate of GIFT is about 27 percent per transfer. Pregnancy may be detected with blood or urine tests ten to twelve days after the procedure. If pregnancy does not occur, the procedure may be repeated in three months. The possible complications of this technique include miscarriage and ectopic pregnancy (pregnancy occurring outside the uterine cavity).

ZYGOTE INTRAFALLOPIAN TRANSFER (ZIFT)

Zygote intrafallopian transfer is an alternative to GIFT, used if there is a question of the sperm's ability to fertilize the egg, due to either a low sperm count or the quality of the sperm.

With ZIFT, the eggs are retrieved in the same way they are for GIFT; however, the eggs and the sperm are then fertilized in the laboratory. This technique is similar to IVF; the only difference lies in where the embryos are placed after the procedure. In ZIFT, they are surgically placed into the fallopian tubes, and in IVF they are placed into the uterus nonsurgically.

As in the GIFT procedure, the eggs are retrieved via an ultrasound-guided needle aspiration under light sedation in the operating room. There is no surgical incision and no subsequent pain; the woman may go home a few hours afterward. The eggs are fertilized and grow for two days in the laboratory. The woman is readmitted to the hospital for the embryos' transfer into her fallopian tubes, a minor surgical procedure identical to GIFT. The woman usually stays in the hospital overnight, and the medications and ovulation stimulators are all the same. Placing the embryos in the fallopian tubes rather than in the uterus yields a higher success rate for this procedure, about 55 percent.

SPERM WASHING

This is a laboratory technique that separates the sperm from the seminal fluid. Semen is collected at home and brought either to the laboratory or to the physician's office. A routine semen analysis is made to determine the quantity and quality of the sperm. The sperm are then placed into a centrifuge (a device that spins test tubes at high speeds and separates the sperm from the seminal fluid), diluted in a culture medium in the presence of antibiotics, and then centrifuged again and incubated. When the woman ovulates, the sperm is placed in her. Sperm washing is extremely important for the new technologies such as IVF and GIFT, as it enhances the sperm's ability to fertilize the egg.

Studies have shown that sperm washing helps to improve the sperm number and the quality of sperm movement while increasing the percentage of sperm moving. The procedure is used for situations in which the man has a low sperm count, the woman has poor cervical mucus (washed sperm easily penetrates the cervical mucus), or sperm antibodies are present. It is also recommended for those couples who have been unsuccessful with other infertility treatments. The procedure has many advantages, including its low cost and the ease with which it is done.

CRYOPRESERVATION

Cryopreservation involves fertilizing all the eggs gathered during in vitro fertilization but transferring only some of the embryos to the uterus. The remaining embryos may be frozen in case pregnancy does not occur with the first try or if the husband wants to maintain possible fertility following a vasectomy or certain medical treatments. When used for the treatment of infertility, this method spares women from having to repeat the egg-retrieval procedure. The embryo itself is placed in a special cryoprotectant, or antifreeze, solution and sucrose. The cryoprotectant insulates the cells and protects them from damage. The embryos are then aspirated into a small plastic freezing straw and the straw is sealed at both ends. The temperature is lowered at a very controlled and slow rate to about –30°C to –40°C (–22°F to –40°F). It is then kept in a large tank of liquid nitrogen. The success rate is approximately 60 percent. In other words, 40 percent of the embryos that are frozen do not survive the freezing process, though it is usually the healthy ones that do survive.

EMBRYO TRANSFER OR EGG DONATION

This alternative is used when the woman is incapable of producing viable eggs or if in vitro fertilization was unsuccessful. This is a realistic alternative for a woman who, after menopause, decides that she wants to become pregnant. While age may rob a woman of viable eggs, it doesn't sacrifice the use of her uterus, as long as she has access to eggs.

A female donor volunteers to become inseminated with the male's sperm. Fertilization occurs in the female volunteer. The infertile woman, in the meantime, is prescribed hormones to prepare her uterus for implantation. If pregnancy occurs, the fertilized embryo is removed from the volunteer and immersed in a protein-enriched culture fluid. It is then placed in a catheter attached to a special syringe, the catheter is passed through the infertile woman's cervix, and the embryo is inserted into the uterus. The woman is advised to remain in bed for one to twelve hours.

What you must understand about this procedure is that you will be receiving a donor egg. Your baby's genes will be a combination of your husband's genes and those of the woman donating the egg. Ideally, you should know the donor. If you don't, many ethical questions could be raised, such as "Whose baby is it?"

This has prompted physicians such as Dr. Mark Sauer of the University of Southern California Medical Center in Los

Angeles to ask his patients to search among their younger relatives, friends, or colleagues for someone willing to donate an egg (*Newsweek*, November 1990). In this way, no one is being paid, but rather the donor is donating out of the goodness of her heart, and more important, the recipient knows the donor.

The first embryo transfer was carried out in 1983 by Dr. John Buster, who at that time was at the University of California in Los Angeles. This first attempt was unsuccessful. In January 1984, however, the first baby was born as a result of this procedure. Today, success rates can be as high as 70 percent.

SURROGATE PARENTING

Surrogate parenting is an option when the man is fertile but the woman is not. It may also be appropriate if the woman fears passing on a certain genetic defect. A surrogate is a woman who volunteers to become impregnated with the sperm of the fertile male partner and carries the pregnancy to term. The couple then adopts the newborn child. Surrogates are often found through local organizations. The difference between surrogate parenting and adoption is that the offspring in the former situation has some genetic makeup directly from the father. In most cases, surrogate parenting is considered a last resort after surgery, or if in vitro fertilization and attempts to adopt have proven unsuccessful.

Although surrogate parenting may be difficult emotionally, especially for the woman bearing the child, it is often the only answer for a childless couple. Surrogate parenting also presents many ethical and legal questions, as demonstrated for the first time by the controversial "Baby M" case in New Jersey in 1987. At that time, Mary Beth Whitehead was denied custody of the child she was contracted to bear. She was later granted visitation rights. Whitehead was impregnated through artificial insemination by the husband of the couple who hired her. She was, therefore, the infant's genetic mother.

A more recent case went one step further. Anna Johnson in California was contracted to carry Crispina Calvert's baby for $10,000 and, after the nine months of pregnancy, changed her mind and wanted to keep the baby. The controversy went to court and it was ruled that the biological parents (the Calverts) were to be the parents of the child, although Anna Johnson said she would continue to fight the legal battle to gain custody. In 1992, the U.S. Supreme Court let stand the initial ruling, asserting that Anna Johnson had no rights to the child, and refused to review the case in a later appeal. This ruling only applies in California; however, in general, most states claim that the husband who is living with the woman when she gets pregnant, no matter where she gets the sperm, is the legal father of the child. For the most part, a woman carrying a baby for nine months does not have to give it up without having previously volunteered to do so.

There has been a dramatic increase in surrogate parenting over the past several years. As biotechnology continues to advance, the courts will likely see more cases where they find they have to reinterpret what was once the simple concept of parenthood. Various organizations have formed to guide parents through this process. Creating Families, Inc., for example, provides references for surrogate mothers and specializes in matching mothers with appropriate families.

SURROGATE UTERUS

This is an alternative for a woman who is unable to carry her baby inside of her. The success of this alternative dates back to 1985. Dr. Wolf Utian and Dr. Leon Sheehan from Cleveland, Ohio, reported for the first time that a woman without a uterus was able to have her own genetic child. She had had an emergency cesarean during pregnancy that resulted in a hysterectomy. After this tragedy, a friend agreed to carry her child, serving as the "surrogate uterus" for nine months.

This technique, sometimes known as "host uterus," starts in the same way as in vitro fertilization in that the couple's egg is fertilized in a petri dish. However, when fertilization occurs, the embryo is transferred to another woman, who will attempt to carry the baby to term. The case a few years back of a South African grandmother who carried her daughter's triplets is a perfect illustration of this method. Unlike a baby born through in vitro fertilization, the baby is genetically linked to both the mother and the father, not to the "host woman."

For the most part, it is believed that the surrogate uterus technique is here to stay and that it is morally and ethically less controversial than some of the other recent medical advances. This alternative simply offers an opportunity for a relative or friend to volunteer to give the greatest possible gift to a woman who is unable to carry her own baby.

○

Treatments for infertility are not always successful. Physicians estimate that for about 10 to 15 percent of infertile women the actual cause of infertility is not identified. Throughout your specialist's investigation it is important to keep all your appointments and to try to continue with your life as before. Maintain a regular exercise regime to help cope with the long process and the natural stresses this produces. Speak to other couples in a similar situation to learn how they are coping and what they are learning from their investigations. It's important not to hesitate to ask questions of your specialist and others—there is no such thing as a stupid question. Above all, keep your spirits up and try at all times to maintain a positive attitude.

Here are some lighthearted hints to help you keep things in perspective:

You know it's going to be a bad day when . . .

1. You put the wrong end of your basal thermometer in your mouth.

2. Your infertility specialist posts the following sign in his office: "We only accept cash for visits and tests. Please pay before leaving."

3. You are taking a semen sample in for analysis and a policeman stops you for speeding and asks you what's in the jar.

4. Your new puppy chews up three months' worth of basal metabolic temperature charts.

5. On the day of your artificial insemination, the doctor cancels because his wife just had twins.

6. The country from which you are adopting a baby has a major military coup and all travel in and out of the country grinds to a halt.

7. The only seat on the bus is beside a very pregnant woman with a cute two-year-old squirming on what's left of her lap.

8. Your Clomid prescription comes in a bottle with a child-proof cap.

9. You start dating your reports at work with the day of your menstrual cycle.

10. You see a "60 Minutes" film crew and Dan Rather entering your adoption agency.

11. You go into your crowded neighborhood pharmacy for BBT supplies and the cashier yells to the druggist at the other end of the store, "Where are the basal thermometers and what the hell are they?"

12. Your house guests mistake the 24-hour urine collection in the refrigerator for cider.

13. In the middle of your hysterosalpingogram, you hear the radiologist say "Oops."

14. Your adopted child comes home with a biology assignment to plot his/her family tree.

15. Your employer calls you in to discuss your bi-weekly absences for "death of a loved one" for the past year and a half.

16. You go into a drugstore to buy a BBT chart and the pharmacist winks suggestively.

(Courtesy of Resolve, Inc.)

Chapter 4

———————— O ————————

High-Risk Factors
Before Pregnancy

HIGH-RISK PREGNANCY: AN INTRODUCTION

A high-risk pregnancy is one that endangers the health and possibly the lives of the mother and her unborn baby. About 15 to 20 percent of all pregnant women have some type of difficulty with their pregnancy. Although sophisticated medical technologies have helped, problem pregnancies are never easy for the mother, the baby-to-be, or the family. They are stressful, and the long road to a healthy birth may be strewn with obstacles.

Your physician may tell you either early or later in your pregnancy that you will have a problem pregnancy. When you are told does not indicate the extent of your risk. For example, a woman over the age of thirty-five will probably be concerned all through her pregnancy that everything is all right, though she may actually be at less risk than an obese younger woman who is told in her thirty-fourth week that she has high blood pressure.

When there is a likelihood that yours will be a high-risk pregnancy because of a preexisting problem, your physician will do a complete physical examination, record your medical history, and then inform you of the risk involved. Pregnancy may have an adverse effect on your condition and, conversely, the disease may affect the pregnancy and its outcome. Ideally, it is best to consult your physician prior to becoming pregnant in order to be aware of any special precautions.

If you are a woman with a history of infertility problems, you will welcome your physician's special precautions. Holding on to the life of a baby is important to all expectant mothers; it is probably even more important to you.

If you are having a high-risk pregnancy, various types of caregivers may monitor your progress before and during your pregnancy. Some women choose to visit their family doctor—a general practitioner—while others prefer to seek the care of a physician specializing in obstetrics. Others may prefer the care of a nurse-midwife.

Obstetricians/gynecologists are physicians who have had three or more years of specialization following their graduation from medical school. They are board-certified. These are the caregivers most often utilized by women having infertility or high-risk pregnancy problems. Although a general practitioner is qualified to follow a woman through her pregnancy, an obstetrician would have to be called in if the need for a cesarean arose.

OB/GYN nurse practitioners are registered nurses who have completed one or more years of postgraduate education, often having completed a master's degree. These professionals specialize in women's health and are qualified to administer routine prenatal care for uncomplicated pregnancies; they are not licensed to deliver babies. Nurse practitioners tend to use a more holistic approach and work in consultation with a physician when problems arise.

A certified nurse-midwife is a registered nurse who has completed one or more years of midwifery training after graduation and is then certified by the American College of Nurse-Midwives. Midwives are capable of caring for uncomplicated pregnancies and births; however, they often work in consultation with a physician should any complications occur.

Childbirth educators work along with the obstetrical team to teach couples about prenatal care, birth, and, in some cases, parenting. These professionals come from varied backgrounds, and in many cases they are nurse-midwives. Childbirth educators believe in family-centered maternity care and freedom of choice based on knowledge of the alternatives. These professionals are often the ones who teach prenatal classes in your area.

Whether you decide to seek the care of a specialist or not, you need to understand your caregiver's plan. Here are some questions you may want to ask:

○ Do you routinely use ultrasound? For what reasons?

○ Do you believe in vaginal birth after cesarean?

O What percentage of your patients have an episiotomy?

O What happens if I have a problem at night or on the week-end? Whom do I call?

O Who covers for you when you are unavailable?

O If I go into preterm labor, what drugs or interventions do you prescribe?

O Will my partner be able to participate in the birth?

O Do you believe in delivering breech babies vaginally?

O How many deliveries have you done in the past twelve months? How many of those were cesareans?

O How do you feel about pain relief during labor?

O Under what conditions do you induce labor?

O Do you believe in hormone therapy for threatened miscarriage?

O What do you recommend for bleeding during pregnancy?

O When is your vacation? If you don't know now, will you tell me in advance? Will I have the opportunity to meet your replacement?

O Do you recommend vitamin supplementation? When and why?

O What dietary recommendations do you have for me?

O What are your fees? How do you handle insurance claims?

There are two types of high-risk pregnancies—those related to chronic conditions of the mother and those stemming from complications with the pregnancy itself. Some women have both problems. In the balance of this chapter we will discuss the problems that may arise due to diseases, illnesses, physiological conditions, and inherited risk factors in the mother.

CHRONIC CONDITIONS OF THE MOTHER

A History of Miscarriage

Miscarriages occur in approximately 15 to 20 percent of all pregnancies within the first five months of pregnancy—most often in the first three months. One woman described her experience:

I vividly remember just having finished the first trimester. It was my second pregnancy, and for me the first three months is always the worst time. I am one of those people who gets extremely nauseated and feels faint half of the time. I saw my obstetrician at about twelve weeks and she was unable to find a fetal heart rate. She recommended having an ultrasound, but I felt it was too early to start with tests. The following week I started bleeding and saw my obstetrician again, and that's when we decided to do an ultrasound. I was shocked—the report showed that there was no fetus. As hard as it was, I went home, only to return a few weeks later to have a D&C.

About 85 percent of miscarriages are due to a genetic disorder in the makeup of the egg that causes the fetus to develop improperly. When this occurs, the embryo disintegrates or is absorbed by the surrounding tissue early in pregnancy. The empty gestational sac is then expelled with the other products of pregnancy (amniotic sac, placenta, amniotic fluid).

Over 60 percent of early pregnancy losses are a result of the products of conception having an extra chromosome or an extra set of chromosomes. The development of an embryo with abnormal chromosomes is most often an accident of that particular pregnancy, but in a small proportion of these instances the condition is inherited.

Some of the causes of miscarriage are discussed more fully below.

Congenital Maternal Anatomical Abnormalities in the Reproductive System These are seen in about one in seven hundred women. Having a congenital abnormality does not mean that you cannot have children, but it may increase your chances of having a miscarriage. Malformations may have occurred during your own fetal development that go unnoticed until you try to have a baby. The malformations may be detected before your pregnancy, but they are usually discovered only when investigative tests are performed after multiple miscarriages. If your physician suspects a malformation in your reproductive system, he or she may order a hysterosalpingogram, or HSG (see chapter 2). This test involves injecting a dye into the uterus through the vagina so that your reproductive system is highlighted when an X-ray is taken.

Anatomical malformations that may trigger a miscarriage include a septate uterus with one cervix, a double uterus with two cervixes, and an incompetent cervix. If you have an incompetent cervix, you may experience a painless miscarriage between the twelfth and twentieth weeks of your pregnancy. A woman with a septate uterus will have a miscarriage associated with discomfort. (These conditions are discussed in detail below.) Another type of structural problem, which may not be congenital, is uterine fibroids (myomas). These are noncancerous growths in the muscle layer of the wall of the uterus that make it difficult for the egg to implant itself. Yet another structural cause of miscarriage is Asherman's syndrome, characterized by scar tissue inside the uterus from overly vigorous D&Cs or from an infection following an abortion.

Bacterial and Viral Infections Infections such as rubella or German measles, active herpes simplex, chlamydia, and cytomegalovirus may affect fetal development and result in miscarriage. At the beginning of your pregnancy you will probably have a test for rubella. However, if you are not immune to German measles and are considering pregnancy, it is a good idea to get vaccinated and then wait three months before trying to conceive.

Pregnant women are prone to vaginal infections. If you are pregnant and have a vaginal infection it is important to have it treated promptly, because the effects on the fetus are still unknown. Treatments with creams and suppositories are usually very successful. Signs of vaginal infection include genital itching, unusual vaginal odor or discharge, and discomfort or a burning feeling during urination.

Maternal Diseases Diabetes, hypertension, thyroid imbalance, sickle-cell anemia, and autoimmune disorders, if not adequately controlled, may result in the loss of a fetus. I will discuss these in more detail later in the chapter.

Women with systemic lupus erythematosus, an autoimmune disease, have an increased incidence of miscarriage, especially if the disease is not in remission. Some women's bodies may respond to the new fetus as a foreign object and reject it. One woman who had six miscarriages before it was learned that she had lupus says,

> I'm glad we decided to start having a family soon after we got married, because only after six miscarriages and one stillbirth did doctors realize what was wrong with me. Autopsies showed that my placenta was completely disintegrated. Finally, my obstetrician prescribed prednisone early in pregnancy to prevent my placenta from disintegrating. It was a long time coming, but it was worth every minute, as I am enjoying my five-year-old daughter so much.

Hormonal Imbalances Hormonal imbalances may be another cause of miscarriage, although some authorities admit that there is a great deal of uncertainty about the relationship between hormonal imbalance and miscarriages. Some sources believe that inadequate progesterone production, or corpus luteum deficiency, may result in early miscarriage. The corpus luteum is the empty follicle that has released the egg. If conception occurs, it serves as a temporary endocrine gland that secretes progesterone, the hormone that thickens the lining of the uterus in preparation for the egg's implantation. When progesterone levels are too low the egg has difficulty implanting itself in the uterine wall, or the pregnancy is not maintained until the developing placenta makes its own hormones.

In some instances, spotting in the early stages of pregnancy may indicate a hormonal deficiency during the implantation period. If a blood test indicates that your progesterone level is low, your specialist may give you progesterone suppositories, vaginal cream, or injections, either for the duration of your luteal phase or in two injections spaced two weeks apart. The injections, often given in the gluteal (buttock) muscles, may be painful because of their oil base. The causes of a decreased progesterone level have not yet been established.

Some authorities believe that adrenal gland problems and a decrease in the secretion of thyroid hormones may also cause miscarriages. Routine blood tests done early in the pregnancy and yearly physical examinations help in identifying hormonal imbalances.

Amniocentesis and Chorionic Villi Sampling (CVS) Although the benefits of these tests often outweigh the risks, in rare instances they can cause miscarriage. Performing amniocentesis and CVS early in the pregnancy is thought to carry a slightly higher risk; however, results tend to fluctuate from medical center to medical center. Couples should consult their caregiver before making the decision to incorporate these procedures as part of the mother's prenatal testing.

Anesthesia The use of anesthesia may be a factor in miscarriage. A recent Canadian study showed that the miscarriage rate was 1.58 times the normal population risk when procedures using general anesthesia were done during either the first or second trimester. The researchers recommended that elective surgery scheduled for pregnant women be either postponed or canceled.

Chromosome Problems In some couples, less than 5 percent, miscarriage may occur recurrently. In this case, there may be a chromosomal problem in one parent in which the chromosomes are arranged abnormally. In general, the parent seems healthy with no signs of genetic problems. However, the unbalanced combinations of rearranged chromosomes present at the time of conception may result in miscarriage. This is one reason for the importance of having genetic counseling following recurrent miscarriages.

Antiphospholipid Antibodies Recurrent miscarriages may also be caused by the presence of certain antibodies. A simple blood test may be performed to catch the problem early. Treatments include aspirin and steroids.

Once a woman has had a miscarriage there is a 15 to 20 percent chance that she will miscarry again. Miscarriages are difficult emotionally, especially if you have been trying to have a baby for a long time. Some women who have had a miscarriage say that they find it hard seeing babies without bursting into tears. Adjusting to the loss often takes time and a great deal of support. (See chapter 9 for more discussion on miscarriage.)

Incompetent Cervix

This is a rare condition characterized by very weak cervical tissue that literally lets the baby "fall" from the womb during the second trimester. It is sometimes associated with a uterine abnormality called a septate uterus (uterus divided into two compartments) and a history of repeated miscarriages. If you have an incompetent cervix, chances are you will miscarry without noticeable pain. In fact, you probably will not know you have an incompetent cervix until you miscarry once or twice after the first trimester. Only then will your physician suspect a problem. If a woman has had previous surgery to her cervix and a problem is already suspected, a physician may perform an ultrasound to measure the patient's cervical length. This will determine if the following treatment is necessary.

The treatment for an incompetent cervix is the surgical placement of a suture or cerclage (McDonald procedure) around the cervix to keep it closed. This procedure is usually done between the twelfth and eighteenth weeks. If you start dilating prior to the twelfth week or have a history of very early miscarriage, your physician may decide to do the procedure earlier. The surgery is often done safely under regional anesthesia, although some physicians choose general anesthesia. Because the surgery is so short, there is little risk of anesthesia adversely affecting your baby. It may be followed by a day or so of hospitalization. This procedure has shown a success rate of 85 to 90 percent.

One woman describes her experience:

I had three healthy children when I became pregnant with my fourth. Right from the start this pregnancy was quite different from the others. I was plagued with cramps, spotting, and nausea. By three months I was quite concerned, as it felt more like the end of pregnancy than the beginning. By four and a half months we were in real trouble. One day I phoned my husband at work because I was bleeding quite heavily and the cramping was more severe. I went to the emergency department and my ultrasound showed that the baby was alive and well. It was thought that the bleeding was caused by a polyp on my cervix, and my ligaments were bothering me.

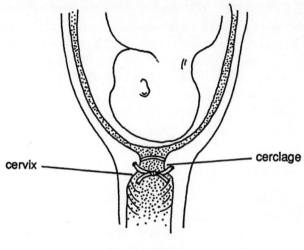

Cervical Suture

I went home and that night was awakened at 2:00 a.m. by intense cramping. I wasn't bleeding, but the cramping was so intense that I went to the hospital. I lost that baby and soon after it was decided I had developed an incompetent cervix. I was relieved to learn this, and very soon after I became pregnant once again and had a cervical suture placed at ten weeks. We didn't want to take any more chances.

Following the suture placement you will be advised to stay in bed, to avoid sexual relations, and to seek domestic assistance. A uterine relaxant may be prescribed in conjunction with bed rest. It is important for you not to lift anything heavy, since this may cause undue pressure on your cervix. Some women relieve even mild pressure on the cervix by placing a pillow underneath the mattress, elevating the foot of the bed. My physician recommended that I elevate my feet above my pelvis to avoid any unnecessary pressure on the cervical suture line. I found this position to be very soothing.

The earlier the suture placement is done, the higher the success rate. Most physicians prefer not to do it prior to the twelfth week because of the risk of natural miscarriage due to an inadequate egg; such miscarriages usually occur before the twelfth week.

The suture usually remains in place until the thirty-seventh week or the onset of labor, at which point your physician will arrange its removal in the office. If you have been taking a uterine relaxant, you will be advised to discontinue it at this time. Some women become frightened when they discontinue their uterine relaxant, thinking that they will go into immediate labor. In most cases, however, labor does not ensue. In some cases, a cesarean may be scheduled for other reasons, while in other cases the woman may continue the pregnancy for anywhere from one or two days to three weeks.

Septate Uterus

A septate uterus is a rare congenital abnormality resulting in a tissue membrane (septum) dividing the uterus into two separate cavities. Sometimes the uterus is divided into two compartments (septate); sometimes it is forked (bicornate). Some physicians recommend surgery to unite the parts of the uterus; this increases the surface area of the uterus, thereby giving the fetus more room to grow. This surgery, however, has its risks, including hemorrhage and, in extreme cases, a hysterectomy if the surgery fails. Some physicians may recommend repeated pregnancies in spite of the risk of miscarrying, in the hope that each pregnancy will stretch the uterus to make it adequate to carry a baby to term. Surgery is used as last resort when the woman has had repeated miscarriages and has become discouraged.

Advanced Age

Some believe that being over the age of thirty-five places you in a high-risk category. While there are certain exceptions, viewing the thirty-five-years-and-over category in this way simply alerts professionals that problems may occur. Many women are choosing to have children later in life, because they want either to develop a career or to ensure a loving relationship with a man. One study that examined the experience of a first pregnancy after the age of thirty-five found that women in that age group want to find the "right time" to become pregnant. Having developed a career and a certain amount of financial security gives women a sense of accomplishment before beginning a family.

Women who choose to start a family after the age of thirty-five may take longer to become pregnant. Fertility tends to decline with age; the chance of conceiving decreases the longer the woman waits.

Women who become pregnant over the age of thirty-five also tend to view pregnancy differently. They may be highly conscious about their pregnancy. Their mature outlook and experience have a definite positive effect on their pregnancy. According to Dr. George Huggins of Francis Scott Key Medical Center in Baltimore, "Today, the female consumer is much more savvy than she was years ago; most of those I see over the age of thirty-five have been very prepared for pregnancy. In addition, the thirty-seven-year-old, for example, is much more attuned, in contrast to the average twenty-year-old, who subconsciously makes the assumption that all will be well."

Studies indicate that mature mothers have increased chances of having various health problems that may complicate their pregnancy. For example, a first-time mother over the age of thirty-five has a greater risk of pregnancy-related problems such as preeclampsia, labor difficulties, and genetic defects such as Downs syndrome (see chapter 14). If you are over thirty-five and pregnant, the best advice is to enjoy your pregnancy. Chances are that it will be uneventful, but it is a good idea to discuss any concerns you may have with your caregiver. If you have any preexisting medical problems, alert your obstetrician before pregnancy. Decide with him or her what extra precautions, if any, you will take. Amniocentesis is sometimes recommended if you are over the age of thirty-five. If you would like to have this test and your physician does not mention it, you should ask.

Diabetes

Diabetics have a metabolic disorder characterized by the inability to produce adequate amounts of insulin, an enzyme needed to help the body use glucose (sugar) for energy. The more severe cases of diabetes are treated with insulin injections, while the milder forms are treated with a special diet and/or blood-sugar-reducing (diabetic) pills. Approximately 4 percent of pregnant women are diabetics. The effect of diabetes on pregnancy depends on the severity of the woman's condition: in general, the younger a woman is when she develops diabetes, the more severe it is. Many diabetic mothers have successful pregnancies, but they need careful monitoring because diabetes is often difficult to control during pregnancy.

During pregnancy women are usually tested for diabetes between twenty-six and twenty-eight weeks. Some health care providers test all women, while others only test those at risk. Risk factors include family history, sugar in the urine, increased weight gain, or an increase in amniotic fluid.

About 3 to 5 percent of pregnant women develop something called "gestational diabetes" as a result of their pregnancy. Gestational diabetes is most commonly found among women over the age of twenty-five or in those carrying a large baby, and it may be detected in routine blood tests in the latter part of pregnancy. It can develop in women who gain excessive weight during pregnancy or those who have a family history of diabetes.

Treatment usually involves dietary changes and in some cases insulin injections. The diet is carefully structured, with six meals daily, including three regular meals and three snacks. A diabetics nurse will instruct you on how to test your own blood sugar level. You should also expect to see your physician about every other week, and a meeting with a nutritionist may also be recommended.

If you keep your regular appointments with your physician, chances are that your diabetes will remain under control. If you do not, however, you run the risk of uncontrolled diabetes, which can lead to complications such as kidney problems, placental insufficiency, preeclampsia, and ketoacidosis. It may also result in having a very large baby. Diabetics are more prone to having excessive amniotic fluid (polyhydramnios), vaginal infections, urinary tract infections, stillbirths, and babies born with congenital abnormalities. You should take careful note of your baby's movements and report anything out of the ordinary. A fetal movement rate of ten kicks every two hours in the hour after eating, from twenty-eight weeks onward, is generally considered healthy.

Sometimes it is necessary for diabetic women to have a cesarean birth, either because of complications related to diabetes or because the baby is too big to pass through the birth canal. Today, however, these problems are rare, especially if the woman has been receiving good prenatal care and diabetes was identified. If you are a diabetic, your baby will probably be carefully monitored after birth to ensure that it is in good health.

Risk factors for Developing Diabetes in Pregnancy

○ Excessive amniotic fluid

○ Diabetes in the family

○ Previous baby with a congenital abnormality

○ Previous delivery of a large baby

○ Diabetes in a previous pregnancy

○ Preeclampsia with pregnancy

○ Previous premature birth

○ Previous stillbirth

○ Previous unexplained newborn death

○ Hypertension

○ Frequent urinary tract/vaginal infections

○ Weighing over two hundred pounds

Thyroid Disease

The thyroid is an endocrine gland located at the front of the neck. It secretes hormones essential to a balanced metabolism. If the thyroid is not working properly, it may be either overactive (hyperthyroidism) or underactive (hypothyroidism).

Hyperthyroidism affects about 0.5 percent of pregnant women. Women with this problem risk having low-birth-weight babies. Hyperthyroidism must be treated with medication, and your physician will monitor you closely during your pregnancy. Hypothyroidism rarely occurs in pregnant women because it tends to be associated with infertility. The condition is treated with thyroid replacements, such as synthroid. If it is left untreated a miscarriage may occur because the fetus depends upon the mother's thyroid activity early in pregnancy.

Epilepsy

Epilepsy is characterized by recurrent seizures brought on by an abnormality of the neurological system. This condition is the most common preexisting neurological disorder among pregnant women, affecting 0.3 percent of all pregnant women. It is estimated that nearly one million American women of childbearing age have epilepsy.

Studies indicate that the hormonal and metabolic changes occurring during pregnancy render the epileptic woman more prone to seizures. Seizures are treated with antiepileptic medications, which in some instances may cause certain fetal malformations. However, more than 90 percent of women on antiseizure medication have normal babies. Most doctors recommend taking large doses of folic acid (.8mg) before conception to help reduce the risk of fetal malformations.

If you are epileptic and are planning to have a child, you should discuss with your physician the best plan for you. If you have not had a seizure for a long time, your physician may try under careful supervision to withdraw the medication for a few months to test your tolerance. If your medication is withdrawn, you will probably be closely monitored during your pregnancy just in case seizures reoccur. If you do have a seizure, your physician should be notified immediately. Seizures interfere with the fetal oxygen supply, which could jeopardize your baby's well-being. Those close to you should be prepared to answer certain questions, such as when it happened, how long it lasted, what type of movements you had, if you were able to speak, and whether you slept afterward.

Systemic Lupus Erythematosus (SLE or Lupus)

Lupus is a chronic inflammatory disease of many systems in the body, occurring predominantly in young women. It affects approximately one in seven hundred women between the ages of fifteen and sixty-four, the onset usually occurring before menopause. The disease may begin abruptly, accompanied by fever and signs of infection, or it may exist unnoticed for months. Sensitivity to light, joint pain, a butterfly rash on the face, fatigue, and weight loss are common. The disease is characterized by flare-ups and is diagnosed by physical examination and blood tests. Treatment is usually with prednisone and azathioprine (Imuran).

Today, there is more hope for women with lupus who want to become pregnant. With optimal care and close supervision, these women are bearing healthy babies. The best time for a woman with lupus to become pregnant is when the disease has been in remission for six months or more. This minimizes the stress on you as well as minimizing your baby's exposure to medications.

In general, the effect of lupus on pregnancy is largely dependent upon the phase in which pregnancy occurs (flare-up or remission). If you are in an active stage of lupus, it may flare up during pregnancy. Most symptoms, such as skin rashes and joint swelling, rarely lead to any permanent damage to the fetus. However, the fetus should be closely monitored for any heart abnormalities, such as heart block, often associated with babies of mothers who have lupus. If heart block is detected, it may be treated with steroid drugs during pregnancy. Babies born with heart block and no other heart problem will do well but will require a pacemaker when they reach their teens.

If you want to become pregnant and have lupus, your physician may prescribe the steroid prednisone and a low dosage of aspirin prior to conception in order to minimize the complications of lupus. Some women have to take prednisone and azathioprine (Imuran) during pregnancy. To date, these have not been associated with birth defects.

The incidence of miscarriage for women with lupus is about 25 percent, and therefore these women are carefully monitored during their pregnancy. One woman with eight pregnancy losses and one child describes her experience with lupus:

Had I known that I had lupus when I became pregnant, it would have been a lot easier. The doctors kept telling me that miscarriage is so common and that I should try again. Being the trusting person that I am, I followed their advice. It wasn't until I had miscarried the fifth time that I decided to change doctors. That doctor began doing tests on me because former autopsies of the fetuses showed that each time the placenta began to disintegrate. After many tests, I found out that I had a form of lupus that becomes very active during pregnancy. I was prescribed cortisone, which helped me. Now whenever I speak to women who miscarry, I encourage them to seek another medical opinion. I don't believe that there is such a thing as a miscarriage without a cause.

Heart Disease

Between 0.5 and 2 percent of pregnant women develop heart disease. A previous episode of rheumatic fever is responsible for about 50 percent of heart problems in pregnant women. Other related ailments are heart-valve problems, congenital heart disease, and abnormal heartbeats. The extra weight and water retention common in pregnancy make the heart work that much harder, and your physician will want to observe you carefully to ensure that you are not subjecting it to excessive stress. If you are symptom-free, it is likely that your pregnancy will have no complications. However, if you have pain, discomfort, difficulty breathing at night or while lying down, and dizziness after activity—that is, symptoms arising after little or no exertion—then you may have a difficult pregnancy.

Although treatment varies depending upon your condition, your doctor will probably suggest a diet with supplemented iron and folic acid (see chapter 6). Medications such as furosemide, digoxin, propranolol, quinidine, heparin, or norpace are sometimes given, with caution. You may be advised to stay in bed in order to avoid unnecessary strain on your heart. Your physician will also probably recommend that you see a cardiologist for a more complete evaluation. Take it easy and avoid any needless stress.

Other Problems

You may have a history of other medical problems that may place your pregnancy in a high-risk category. If you have a special problem, remember to ask your physician how your pregnancy will be affected and what he or she recommends for you. Physicians have many patients and many things on their mind, and they cannot be expected to remember everything. Reminding your physician of your important medical details is your responsibility—and always remember to mention any medications you are taking.

Chapter 5

──────── O ────────

High-Risk Complications During Pregnancy

In addition to the type of chronic problems discussed in the last chapter, there are a number of conditions that can be especially dangerous if they develop during your pregnancy. Some of them, like hypertension or the HIV virus, can be serious and life-threatening at any time. Others, like urinary tract infections, are dangerous because of the threat they pose to the fetus developing within you. A third group are conditions specifically associated with the pregnancy. The most commonly encountered complications—and some of the more serious ones—are discussed below.

HYPERTENSION

Hypertension is a condition in which the person has a higher blood pressure than that considered normal for his or her age and weight. There are two types of hypertension during pregnancy: pregnancy-induced hypertension (PIH), and the hypertension that existed before the woman became pregnant. Hypertension affects approximately 7 percent of pregnant women in the United States, most of whom have pregnancy-induced hypertension. It is most common in women who are pregnant for the first time and are over the age of thirty-five or under the age of eighteen. If you are over thirty-five, have a family history of hypertension, are diabetic, are overweight, have kidney disease, or are carrying multiple fetuses, you are at greater risk of developing high blood pressure.

If blood pressure is not maintained at normal levels, it may result in intrauterine growth retardation, premature birth, or stillbirth. However, today hypertension can be successfully treated if it is detected early. The treatment primarily involves teaching a woman how to keep her blood pressure down without the use of medications. Women are often told to lie on their side whenever possible and to limit salt products in their diet. Water retention can cause the blood pressure to rise and therefore should be avoided. Avoid foods such as potato chips, pickles, smoked meats, and carbonated beverages. A high-protein diet may also be recommended to replace the protein lost in the urine.

Bed rest (see chapter 8) is sometimes recommended, usually along with at least eight to twelve hours of sleep each night. An afternoon nap will also help to relax you and minimizes the chances of overworking the heart. Smoking is especially discouraged for those with elevated blood pressure, because the combined effect of smoking and hypertension results in poor blood circulation to the heart.

TOXEMIAS

The word toxemia comes from the Greek words *toxikon*, poison, and *haima*, blood, and refers to problems related to hypertension occurring during pregnancy. The exact cause of the condition is unknown. The problems usually occur in the later part of pregnancy, after twenty-four weeks, when you begin putting on more weight and have a tendency toward water retention. There are two types of toxemia during pregnancy: preeclampsia and eclampsia.

Preeclampsia is the milder form. It is related to inadequate kidney function and is characterized by hypertension, water retention (edema), and protein in the urine (proteinuria). It develops in approximately 7 percent of pregnant women, usually first-time mothers. It usually occurs after the twentieth week of gestation but may occur before that, brought on by other ailments. The effects range from mild to severe. Symptoms include headaches, blurred vision, epigastric (upper abdomen) pain, and unusual swelling of the face and lower legs. Some complain that their hands feel as if they are ballooning.

Treatment for preeclampsia depends upon its severity. Bed rest is usually recommended, as well as lying on your side, which helps to increase the fetus's blood supply. Dietary changes, as mentioned earlier for hypertension, are also recommended.

Women are usually monitored closely with blood tests and non-stress tests (NSTs). Sometimes hospitalization is necessary, and occasionally medicines are prescribed to prevent seizures or early labor. Some women carrying multiple fetuses may be advised to go on bed rest in the latter part of their pregnancy.

One mother recalls her preeclampsia in the latter part of her pregnancy:

> I'll never forget how swollen my hands were. I had been married for five years and my wedding ring grew so tight that I had to have it cut off—it was causing my finger to turn blue. I couldn't even open the door to get the newspaper from outside. I often wondered what I would do if we had a fire in the duplex—how would I escape? My doctor treated my problem by putting me on bed rest for the last two months of my pregnancy. It managed to keep my blood pressure down without the use of medications. I was also very strict about my diet. The hardest part, however, was after waking up in the morning. My hands and feet were so stiff that I had to wait an hour before I was even able to dress myself . . . when I finally did, gee, did I look funny in my husband's running pants and size 12 slippers! Anyway, it was all worthwhile because I had two healthy seven-pound boys at thirty-six weeks.

Eclampsia is serious and is the result of untreated preeclampsia. It is sometimes seen in those who received inadequate prenatal care. It is characterized by grand mal convulsions, coma, hypertension, edema, and proteinuria. There is a possibility of death for both mother and baby, so early delivery is often recommended. Today, eclampsia is rare because regular prenatal visits detect early changes and treatment is initiated immediately.

HYPEREMESIS GRAVIDARUM

Many women have occasional nausea and vomiting associated with early mornings in the first trimester. Having small, frequent meals and only drinking liquids between meals is usually helpful in relieving these symptoms. However, if the symptoms go beyond mild nausea, the rare condition of hyperemesis gravidarum is usually suspected. This condition is characterized by persistent nausea and vomiting that usually begins in the first trimester.

The symptoms of hyperemesis gravidarum are weight loss, dehydration, and imbalances of the body's electrolytes, such as potassium and sodium. Hospitalization is often necessary to provide intravenous nourishment and psychological support. Some sources indicate that this condition may be associated with increased levels of chorionic gonadotropin hormones, the hormones secreted by the placenta in pregnancy and present in the urine of pregnant women. These hormones are the indicators of pregnancy in pregnancy tests. They alter the body's metabolism, which may result in a slowing down of digestion. Very severe vomiting and nausea in pregnancy has also been associated with hydatiform mole (discussed later).

GALLSTONES

The gallbladder is a sac located under the edge of the liver. Its role is to store bile, which aids in digestion. Those who develop gallstones are frequently overweight and consumers of large amounts of fatty or highly seasoned foods. Gallstones (cholelithiasis) are more common in pregnant women, and pregnancy may also exacerbate the problem, leading to an inflammation of the gallbladder (cholecystitis).

The symptoms of gallstones include a sudden aching pain in the upper right part of your abdomen, sometimes radiating to the back and shoulder. It usually occurs after eating, especially after eating fatty foods. The pain or sense of fullness lasts fifteen to sixty seconds. If you have gallstones, your physician may simply suggest a change in diet and may recommend pain-relieving medications, such as meperidine or morphine. Surgery may be necessary in certain situations, and the risks are similar to those for other problems in pregnancy—preterm labor and miscarriage.

APPENDICITIS

This inflammation of the appendix occurs in approximately one in every one thousand pregnancies. Most cases of sudden appendicitis occur within the first six months of pregnancy. One problem with appendicitis in pregnancy is that it may be difficult to diagnose in time; the physician may have difficulty doing an adequate physical examination. There is a chance of the appendix rupturing, which in some cases causes a life-threatening situation. For unknown reasons, pregnant women are two to three times more likely to suffer a ruptured appendix than those who are not pregnant.

If you have sharp pain in the lower right part of your abdomen, you should see your physician immediately. In pregnant women, the pain may also be identified in the right upper part of the abdomen because the uterus has pushed your abdominal contents upward. Often this pain is confused with gallbladder pain in the pregnant woman. Ruptured or not, the appendix is usually removed—the risks of surgery are less than those for a ruptured appendix. Some doctors recommend waiting until after delivery for removal, but this decision is highly individual.

THROMBOEMBOLISM

This is a condition in which a blood vessel becomes blocked by a clot that has traveled through the bloodstream from some other site. This is relatively rare during pregnancy but is more common in those who are relatively immobile. What happens is that blood pools in your lower legs, making a perfect environment for blood-clot formation. This is one good reason to do the passive exercises during bed rest described in chapter 8. Other high-risk situations may predispose a woman to thromboembolism, including abortion, cesarean birth, or pelvic infection following delivery.

In the nonpregnant woman, anti-blood-clotting medications (anticoagulants), such as coumadin, taken orally, are prescribed in order to thin the blood. Sometimes there are side effects from this medication. Heparin, another anticoagulant usually given subcutaneously and intravenously, does not affect the fetus because the heparin molecule is too large to pass through the placenta. If you are not hospitalized, you may be taught how to give yourself heparin injections at home. Minor cases of thromboembolism are usually treated medically. Surgery is saved for those who are in a life-or-death situation.

INFECTIONS

An infection that you may have ignored before pregnancy could be a real danger when you are expecting. All infections pose a potential risk to mother and child. Some common types of infection include kidney/urinary infections, sexually transmitted diseases (syphilis, gonorrhea, herpes, cytomegalovirus, chlamydia), HIV virus, toxoplasmosis, rubella, and chicken pox.

Urinary Tract Infections (UTIs)

Sometimes a urine culture will show bacteria in the urine while the woman does not have the associated symptoms. This is why all pregnant women have routine urine tests early in pregnancy. If an infection is found, it will be treated with oral sulfonamides, ampicillin, or macrodantin. Some women find that regular use of cranberry juice or vitamin C helps make their urine more acidic and therefore helps prevent infection. Whole grains, nuts, and fresh fruits also help acidify the urine. Some herbal teas such as uva ursi, horsetail, shavegrass, cornsilk cleavers, and lemon balm are good for the bladder. However, if you are pregnant you should speak with an herbalist before drinking these teas.

If you have a urinary tract infection, it should be treated as soon as possible. You may have the following signs, which indicate a urinary tract infection: feeling like you have to urinate frequently—and when you go it turns out to be in small amounts—a stinging or burning sensation while you void, discomfort in the kidney region or the lower back, and sometimes blood in the urine (hematuria). Some women are more prone to urinary tract infections than others. The tips below have helped many of my patients in the past.

Preventing Urinary Tract Infections

○ Drink six to eight glasses of water daily.

○ Avoid perfumed toilet papers, soaps, and bubble baths.

○ Avoid feminine hygiene sprays and douches.

○ After intercourse, try urinating and then drink a glass of water.

○ Wash after intercourse.

○ Urinate at the first urge.

○ Treat vaginal infections as soon as symptoms occur.

Kidney Problems

Kidney disease is much more difficult to treat than UTIs. For the most part, however, with prompt diagnosis and treatment most kidney infections will not harm the mother or baby. Kidney problems such as pyelonephritis may occur if a urinary tract infection goes untreated. Kidney infections may also be due to other illnesses, such as diabetes and lupus.

Pyelonephritis

Pyelonephritis is an inflammation of the kidney usually caused by bacteria that have ascended from the bladder after entering through the urethra. It may be caused by an untreated urinary tract infection. If left untreated, it can lead to intrauterine growth retardation and preterm labor.

The symptoms of pyelonephritis include fever, chills, aching lower back, loss of appetite, and nausea/vomiting. Treatment is with intravenous antibiotics in the hospital.

Syphilis

With prenatal screening tests done early in pregnancy, the incidence of syphilis has decreased dramatically over the years. Since the 1940s, the incidence of syphilis has fallen nearly 99 percent. Those who receive inadequate prenatal care are at greatest risk for developing syphilis.

The first stage of this sexually transmitted disease is characterized by a painless chancre that appears between ten and ninety days after exposure and heals within forty days of its appearance. The second stage is characterized by a rash, accompanied by malaise, fever, and aching bones. It is very contagious during this stage, which lasts about three months. The third stage is characterized by latency (no symptoms) as the organism invades other parts of the body. During this stage, a woman can continue to infect her unborn children for up to four years after she initially contracted the disease.

If diagnosed early, treatment with penicillin or erythromycin is very effective. If it is treated prior to sixteen weeks of pregnancy, the mother will be completely cured and the infant will be unaffected.

Those who have not received treatment will bear a baby with syphilis, and it may either die or have serious congenital deformities. It will have a 50 percent chance of death in infancy.

Gonorrhea

Today, gonorrhea is detected during prepregnancy and prenatal screening. Gonorrhea is transmitted through sexual contact. In men, the main symptom is a disturbing burning of the penis with a pus discharge. Women may be free of symptoms and may carry the organism for years without knowing it. Eventually a woman who has the disease develops pelvic inflammatory disease (see chapter 1). Often it is detected when the woman develops otherwise unexplainable arthritis.

If a woman with gonorrhea becomes pregnant, the risks to the fetus include preterm labor, growth impairment, and newborn conjunctivitis between two and seven days after birth. To prevent the latter, the standard practice in North American hospitals is to administer silver nitrate or erythromycin eyedrops to newborns within one hour after birth. Penicillin or spectinomycin are the two most common treatments for gonorrhea. Erythromycin is sometimes given because of the increased chance of chlamydia being present with gonorrhea.

Genital Herpes or Herpes Simplex Type II

This is the most prevalent sexually transmitted disease in the United States. More than thirty million Americans over the age of fifteen (one out of six persons) have it, but most don't develop symptoms. In women, genital herpes is characterized by blisters or ulcers on the genitals lasting one to three weeks. When the ulcers are present, herpes is very contagious. Its most serious aspect, however, is that the disease organism remains dormant between outbreaks. People who come into sexual contact with someone with herpes may unknowingly be infected as well.

It is rare for herpes to be transmitted through the placenta to the fetus. Those who are infected with genital herpes early in pregnancy, during critical periods of fetal development, may have a higher incidence of miscarriage or stillbirth than others. Those infected with herpes after twenty weeks of gestation have a higher incidence of preterm labor and transmission of the virus to the newborn baby. The baby can contract the herpes virus through the birth canal, creating the risk of brain damage, blindness, and death. If there are no lesions, the risk to the baby is low. A cesarean will be done if herpes is active when labor starts, because the herpes virus usually passes from mother to baby when the membranes rupture in labor and/or during vaginal delivery.

Your physician should know if you want to become pregnant and have a history of herpes. Today, only women with lesions are tested. If there is no active infection, the baby may be delivered vaginally.

Cytomegalovirus (CMV)

This is the most common type of uterine viral infection and about six thousand babies each year develop life-threatening complications as a result. CMV is spread by intimate contact with infected body fluids, such as breast milk, cervical mucus, semen, saliva, and urine. For most adults there are no symptoms. For others the symptoms are similar to those of mononucleosis. To date, there is no treatment for CMV. The risk of getting CMV may be minimized by good hand washing and personal hygiene for those who have a great deal of contact with infants and children.

Approximately 10 to15 percent of infants born to women who get CMV in pregnancy suffer mental retardation, a small head, blindness, epilepsy, and other disorders. If the virus is contracted by the baby during delivery the symptoms may not appear for a number of years. Parents may notice hearing difficulties, learning problems, and a high susceptibility to infections in the first two years.

CMV is detected with a blood test, and some institutions do routine blood tests on newborns to detect it. Although the brain

damage is not reversible, the parents can make long-term decisions concerning the child's care and/or prepare for the early
treatment of learning and hearing problems.

Chlamydia

Chlamydia is the most common bacterial STD in the United
States today. About four million new cases occur each year.
Chlamydia is particularly contagious because it is not always
accompanied by symptoms: about 70 percent of women don't
have symptoms. If symptoms are present, they include an inflammation of the urethra (urethritis) in the male, and a vaginal
infection, spotting, urinary urgency and frequency, pain during
sexual intercourse, and malaise in the female. Sometimes these
symptoms lead to PID and possibly to infertility. Unfortunately,
those who are without symptoms are often the ones who spread
this intracellular bacteria. If you do have any of these symptoms
it is important to see your physician so that treatment can be initiated immediately. Diagnosis is made through bacteriologic
exams of urine and vaginal and urethral discharge. Your doctor
may prescribe erythromycin, doxycline, or azithromycin.

Recent research indicates that women with chlamydia are
more likely to have premature delivery or miscarriage. During
vaginal delivery the bacteria is passed on to the fetus, resulting in
newborn conjunctivitis or pneumonia, which begins within a few
days after birth. Conjunctivitis in the newborn can be successfully treated with preventive antibiotic eye ointment.

HIV Infection

HIV (human immunodeficiency virus) is the virus that causes
AIDS, and it may be passed from mother to child during pregnancy. AIDS is a fatal disease that destroys the body's ability to
fight infection. Although in North America it was initially con-
fined largely to homosexual men, it is often found now among
heterosexuals, which means that it may affect a pregnant woman
and her unborn baby.

The number of cases of AIDS has increased dramatically in
the past few years. According to the National Institute of Allergy

and Infectious Diseases, an estimated 33.4 million people world-wide are living with AIDS as of December 1998. AIDS is transmitted by body fluids, such as semen and blood. Those at risk of developing AIDS, such as hemophiliacs, intravenous drug users, prostitutes, homosexuals, and heterosexuals with multiple partners, should be screened for the disease. At the time of this writing, there is still no cure for AIDS, although researchers are working aggressively to find one. Researchers agree that a vaccine for AIDS is still several years away. According to a recent study done by the Centers for Disease Control (CDC) in Atlanta, AIDS is the third leading cause of death among women age twenty-five to forty-four. Approximately eighty thousand new infections occur each year, and women account for more than 22 percent of those cases. Furthermore, the U.S. Department of Health and Human Services and the CDC claim that 80 percent of the cases of AIDS in women are found among women of childbearing age (fifteen to forty-four years of age). About one-fourth of these women were aged twenty to twenty-nine at the time of diagnosis; many were infected as teenagers.

If AIDS is transmitted across the placenta, the baby develops neonatal AIDS. The symptoms may include failure to thrive, enlarged lymph nodes, blood and spleen problems, pneumonia, recurrent infections, and various neurological abnormalities. Unfortunately, if the virus is active, the child will die within one or two years. Others who are simply carrying the virus (testing positive but with no clinical manifestations) have lived for up to eight years.

In an article by Marta Gwinn in the April 1991 issue of the *Journal of the American Medical Association*, it was estimated that eighty thousand American women of childbearing age are actually carrying the HIV virus. If these women get pregnant, approximately 15 to 30 percent of their infants will acquire the virus. The study concluded that in 1990 approximately eighteen hundred babies were born with the HIV virus. According to the March of Dimes Foundation's statistics for 1997, one in twenty-seven hundred babies were born with congenital HIV in the United States. Today, if an HIV-positive mother takes AZT (Zidovudine) during both pregnancy and delivery, the baby's risk of infection may be reduced to 5 percent. Other antiviral drugs may be prescribed with AZT during pregnancy. Nonetheless, preventing the transmission of HIV infection to women and infants remains an urgent public health priority.

Some states already require routine blood testing of pregnant women for AIDS exposure. Beginning in 1991, the Centers for Disease Control in collaboration with state and local health organizations began to strengthen programs to prevent HIV transmission in women. For more information on AIDS in pregnancy, call the National AIDS Information Clearinghouse at 1-800-458-5231. (For other resource groups and associations, see Appendix C.)

TOXOPLASMOSIS

Toxoplasmosis is caused by a parasite found in domestic cat feces, soil, and raw meat. It occurs most frequently in tropical climates. Approximately 15 to 40 percent of American women have been exposed to toxoplasmosis and about 0.6 to 6 out of 1,000 babies have been exposed. The incidence of congenital infection ranges from one in 500 to one in 3,000 deliveries, depending on the part of the country. Fetal blood sampling is sometimes done between twenty and twenty-four weeks to diagnose the presence of congenital infection.

The earlier in the pregnancy that this disease occurs, the more severe is the damage to the fetus. A baby born with this virus is often small and has birth defects. Toxoplasmosis during pregnancy may cause miscarriage, prematurity, stillbirth, or neonatal death. The maternal treatment is with folinic acid, sulfadizine, or pyrimethamine, which can reduce the risk of fetal infection about 50 percent.

Preventing Toxoplasmosis

○ Practice meticulous hand washing during pregnancy, especially after handling cats.

○ Eat only well-cooked meat.

○ Carefully clean counters and utensils after preparing meat.

○ Wash fruits and vegetables well.

○ Wear gloves when gardening.

○ Have another family member change the cat litter box (daily cleaning is recommended).

RUBELLA

Rubella, or German measles, is a highly contagious disease characterized by fever, malaise, and generalized skin rash. The virus multiplies in the upper respiratory tract and enters the bloodstream after seven to ten days. Although some women do not have the typical symptoms, the fetus is quite vulnerable.

About 50 to 80 percent of fetuses are affected by rubella if the mother is exposed during the first trimester. About one-third of these pregnancies end in miscarriage, and two-thirds result in serious congenital abnormalities. About 30 percent of afflicted babies will die within the first four months of life. If they live longer, they may be found to have learning problems. If a mother is exposed in the second or third trimester there is a minimal chance of congenital problems.

The best treatment for rubella during pregnancy is its prevention. Routine prenatal blood tests done early in pregnancy indicate a woman's rubella antibody level. If a woman is susceptible to infection and has been exposed, genetic counseling will provide an option for elective abortion. If you are pregnant and have never had rubella, but are exposed to a child with the disease, you should notify your physician.

The number of rubella cases has decreased dramatically over the past three decades. According to the Centers for Disease Control, from April 1990 to April 1991 there were only 245 reported cases in the United States; in 1989 there were 396 cases. This is a dramatic decrease, as in 1985 there were 604 reported cases, which at that time was the lowest rate since 1966. Today, researchers estimate that 1 in every 100,000 babies will have rubella.

Today, a rubella immunization is administered routinely in early childhood. If you have not had rubella yourself and are not pregnant, it is a good idea to get immunized. The best time to do this is immediately after the start of your menstrual period, so that you can be sure you are not pregnant. You should wait at least three months before trying to become pregnant. If, however, you are pregnant and are not immune, it would be a good idea to be immunized after this pregnancy to avoid problems in future pregnancies.

CHICKEN POX

Chicken pox, or the varicella-zoster virus, is the second most reported infectious disease in the United States. It is characterized by feelings of malaise, headache, fever, and the eruption of crusty pustules on the skin.

According to the March of Dimes, between one and seven of every ten thousand pregnant women get chicken pox. It may have detrimental effects on the developing fetus, especially if it is contracted during the first trimester or in the last few days before birth.

If chicken pox is contracted before the sixteenth week of pregnancy, the baby may suffer severe malformations, usually detected through ultrasound. Some physicians give a solution of immunoglobulin to women exposed to chicken pox in the first or second trimester. It is unclear whether this prevents fetal abnormalities, but it has been shown to prevent complications for the mother. If a mother develops chicken pox during delivery, the baby may develop a rash one to two weeks after the mother's sores appeared.

MULTIPLE PREGNANCY

Multiple pregnancies occur more often than previously thought, about once in every eighty pregnancies. According to the American College of Obstetricians and Gynecologists, the number of twins being born has gone up 33 percent over the last decade. The number of triplets, quadruplets, and other high-order births has gone up 178 percent. Twins are formed from either one egg (identical twins) or two eggs (fraternal twins). Fraternal twins are more common and can be either of the same sex or different sexes.

If there is a history of twins in your family, your chance of having twins is increased. If you have been taking fertility drugs, your chance of multiple pregnancy is also increased. Other persons possibly at risk for twins include those who have recently been on the Pill, those who have undergone IVF (in vitro fertilization) or GIFT (gamete intrafallopian transfer), and those who are over forty and who have had four or more children.

Carrying more than one baby will usually be detected early in pregnancy by ultrasound and by tests that show elevated blood levels of alpha fetoprotein. Two sacs may be seen on the ultrasound as early as six to eight weeks. Your physician may also suspect a multiple pregnancy because of your weight gain and the size of your uterus or because he or she hears two heartbeats. A situation termed "vanishing twin syndrome" sometimes occurs, in which one of the twins is reabsorbed by the mother's body. This usually occurs early in pregnancy, prior to the sixteenth week.

Many women feel perfectly fine during a multiple pregnancy. However, your physician will want to carefully monitor your progress. Most professionals recommend bimonthly checkups for the first half of the pregnancy and weekly checkups thereafter. In addition, you may be advised to increase your nutritional and vitamin intake. You may also be told to curtail strenuous sports and to plan several rest periods during the day. If you have a stressful and tiring job, you might be well advised to take a leave of absence or to decrease your hours to ensure that you get adequate rest.

Bed rest is commonly prescribed for those carrying more than one baby, in order to prevent early labor and delivery. Physicians have differing opinions about when bed rest should start. The most common recommendation, however, is at about the thirtieth week (see chapter 8). Even though bed rest may not be prescribed early in your case, it is especially important that any mother of multiples receive plenty of rest. Ideally, you should rest in a semi-recumbent position or lying down on the left side, as this takes the pressure off your vena cava, the principal vein down your back, which drains blood from the upper part of the body. These rest periods should occur two or three times daily.

The risks associated with multiple pregnancies are much lower than they were years ago. Some problems may arise, but today, with early detection, these are quite manageable. The possible problems include hypertension, anemia, unusual fetal positions, gestational diabetes, stillbirths, smaller babies, and early delivery. Frequent blood-sugar tests will be done to detect diabetes, and your blood pressure will be carefully monitored.

Expect repeat ultrasounds to check the baby's growth, cervical checks, and nonstress tests as part of the standard procedure for monitoring twins. Premature birth is the single most important risk with multiple pregnancies, occurring ten times more often than with singletons. Approximately half of all twins and three-quarters of triplets are born before the thirty-seventh week.

Coping emotionally with a multiple pregnancy may not be easy, especially if there are other children at home or if a multiple pregnancy is learned about late in the pregnancy. Some women react with excitement:

I was absolutely ecstatic when I heard that I was having twins. I already had a three-year-old at home and this did not bother me. I knew when I was only six weeks pregnant that there was a possibility that I would have twins. At three months, the ultrasound showed that there were two amniotic sacs. I was warned about the possibility of having premature babies but was confident that everything would be all right. It sure was—at thirty-eight weeks I gave birth to two healthy seven-pound twins, one girl and one boy.

Other women react with fear and anger:

After two years of infertility work-ups you'd think I would be happy. However, I encountered the opposite reaction. I suddenly didn't want to be pregnant anymore. I cried an awful lot. For financial and emotional reasons, I felt I would be unable to offer my children the best. I always dreamt about cuddling one baby. I never felt happy about having twins—but it was something I grew to accept. My husband, on the other hand, felt the opposite. He was delighted that he too could have the one-on-one relationship with a baby at the same time as me.

The actual adjustment to a multiple pregnancy depends on the individual woman and other factors, including the woman's partner, family, age, economic status, health, and personal philosophy. A very common concern for the couple is the effect on their relationship after two or more babies are born. They may have feelings of inadequacy, of being unable to cope with more than one child. For the most part, extra babies are not planned, although with the advent of ultrasound they may at least be expected. This gives the couple time to prepare as well as to seek outside assistance. Sometimes husbands look forward to the multiple birth, because they know they will be more involved in the early stages, when the woman has to juggle two or more crying babies.

Many couples, however, tend to underestimate the workload involved in caring for more than one baby at a time. The stress may lead to marital problems, depression, and child abuse. If you find you are overstressed, it is important to seek counseling in order to avoid any of these potential side effects of multiple births.

Learning how to ask for help is very important for the mother who is going through a multiple pregnancy. You will need your strength, and a few hours of assistance during the day from a mother's helper or a relative may help you conserve that needed energy. Speaking with other mothers who have had multiple pregnancies may help you gain much-needed perspective. Some local twins clubs have telephone committees that help minimize the sense of isolation experienced by so many new mothers. These women may also be able to advise you on other resources, such as where to get used furniture, strollers, and clothes, because you will have to have double, if not more, of everything. A strong support system is important during these times. At a later date, you might be interested in helping other new mothers.

Unusual Fetal Positions

Most babies move around in the uterus for the first six months but settle into the head-down position by the seventh or eighth month. Sometimes babies may choose the breech position, where their head is up, as though they were sitting inside of you. This occurs in approximately 3 to 4 percent of all deliveries. Some other, rarer positions include shoulder presentation, face presentation, and transverse position.

A breech position may be suspected during one of your routine prenatal visits when your baby is being palpated. It may also be suspected when your baby's heartbeat is heard above your navel rather than below it. Your baby's position may also be identified during ultrasound examination. Women who have a baby in this position often say that they feel the fetus's kicks lower in their abdomen. It is very difficult to have a breech baby vaginally. The safest position for the baby's head is for it to be tucked into its chest. If the baby's head is extended backward and it is delivered vaginally, there is a real risk of damaging the neck and the spine.

The management of breech presentation varies. Some methods are recommended because the mother can do them herself; these are called the positioning methods. In one such method the woman, in her last month of pregnancy, is told to lie on her back on a firm surface with the hips elevated about nine to twelve inches by pillows for about ten minutes, twice daily. It is important that this be done on an empty stomach. If you feel that the baby has turned, this exercise should be discontinued and your health care provider should be notified about the position change. The technique is not always effective.

Some women try unusual yoga positions or standing on their head to help their baby turn. Others advocate maintaining a head-down position, crouching on your hands and knees with your head down and buttocks up, for fifteen minutes twice daily. You should check with your physician prior to performing any of these procedures; they are advised only under careful supervision.

External rotation or version is another way to turn a baby. This method is advocated more and more today in an effort to cut costs and reduce the number of cesarean deliveries. The technique may be used for those at thirty-seven to thirty-nine weeks.

First the baby's position is verified by ultrasound. A medication is given to relax the uterus. The physician or midwife places one hand on your abdomen over the baby's head and the other hand over its buttocks. The hands are moved in opposite directions and the baby is gently stroked to encourage it to change positions. Some caregivers fear rotating, however, because of the risk of the umbilical cord becoming wrapped around the fetus's neck.

Studies vary as to how late in pregnancy the fetus can turn itself. Some claim that the baby may turn itself even after the twenty-eighth week. Timing is very important, because if the rotation is done too far in advance the baby may revert to the breech position by the time of delivery. In addition, if a complication such as abruptio placenta or a change in the baby's heart rate should occur, an emergency cesarean would be necessary, resulting in the delivery of a premature baby. If you have a breech presentation and want to have a vaginal delivery, speak with your physician. He or she may consent with the understanding that you might have to have an emergency cesarean in the event of problems.

BLOOD INCOMPATIBILITIES

If you have a negative Rh (rhesus) factor, your physician will monitor you very closely during your pregnancy. Approximately 15 percent of the population is Rh-negative and about five thousand newborns are afflicted with Rh disease each year. If you are Rh-negative and this is your first pregnancy it will not be a problem, because your blood and your baby's blood rarely mix until pregnancy ends. However, a problem can occur with your second pregnancy.

In your second pregnancy, if you and your baby are Rh-negative, the pregnancy will go well. However, if you are Rh-negative and your baby is Rh-positive there will be a problem unless the situation is detected. As the fetus grows, some of the red blood cells that it produces pass through the placenta into the mother's blood, and her system produces antibodies to the Rh factor. These antibodies recross the placenta and destroy the fetus's red blood cells. The baby is born with abnormal blood cells, a condition called erythroblastosis, which may lead to anemia, jaundice, or both. In very severe cases it may cause stillbirth.

If you are Rh-negative and the father of your fetus is Rh-negative, the fetus will also be Rh-negative and therefore there will be no problem. However, if you are Rh-negative and the father is Rh-positive, the fetus may be Rh-positive.

To prevent any problem from occurring, you will be given an immunizing agent such as RhoGAM, first during your pregnancy between your twenty-eighth and thirty-second week, and then within seventy-two hours after your baby is born. All Rh-negative mothers should receive this injection after every pregnancy, whether it goes to full term or is terminated by abortion or miscarriage.

VAGINAL BLEEDING

Some causes of vaginal bleeding are

o Egg implantation in the uterus

◯ Diminished progesterone

◯ Imminent miscarriage

◯ Incompetent cervix

◯ Placenta previa

◯ Abruptio placenta

Bleeding during pregnancy can be a very frightening and uncertain experience. Anywhere from 25 to 50 percent of pregnant women spot at some time during their pregnancy. The spotting is most often in the first two months of pregnancy, most often between the ninth and twelfth week. Spotting does not necessarily mean that the pregnancy is at risk, but it is always better to be safe than sorry by calling your physician or going to the emergency room at your local hospital.

What is done about your bleeding depends upon what trimester you are in. You may have an internal examination with great caution. Sometimes a speculum is inserted to determine whether the source of bleeding is the cervix, the uterus, or the vagina. If your physician believes that it is inevitable that a miscarriage will occur, then he or she may choose to take a "wait and see" approach. In either case, an ultrasound will be done to detect your baby's status.

What to Do If You Bleed

◯ Phone your physician or nurse-midwife.

◯ Document the amount of bleeding, color of the blood (bright, brownish), and the type of pain (constant, intermittent).

◯ Recall any associated symptoms.

◯ Recall what you were doing when the bleeding began.

◯ If the bleeding is severe and painful, go to the emergency room immediately.

The incidence of significant vaginal bleeding in the last half of pregnancy is about 3 percent, most often due to abnormalities of the placenta. This bleeding is usually intermittent and painless. If you have any bleeding in the last half of your pregnancy, it is important that you go immediately to the hospital. You will be seen by a physician and an ultrasound will probably be done to pinpoint the source of your bleeding.

ABRUPTIO PLACENTA

This is the leading cause of neonatal mortality and requires an emergency cesarean. It occurs once in every eighty-five to twenty births (studies vary). Abruptio placenta is characterized by premature separation of the placenta from the uterus. The separation may be partial or complete. The exact cause is unknown, but some possible related factors include smoking, cocaine use, trauma to the abdomen, short umbilical cord, uterine abnormalities, hypertension, and more than five past pregnancies.

If you have abruptio placenta, you will know that something is happening to you. You may have any of the following symptoms: vaginal bleeding after the twentieth week, decreased fetal movement, and sudden and severe abdominal pain. There may be tenderness when your abdomen is palpated. Because of the threat to both you and your baby, you will be closely monitored. If you have a partial separation, you will be put on complete bed rest in the hospital. Your heart rate and your baby's heart rate will be continuously monitored. If you go into premature labor, you will be given magnesium sulfate to halt labor. If you have a more severe abruptio placenta, delivery by cesarean section may be the only option to save both your lives. One of the risks of a complete abruptio placenta is a possible hysterectomy.

PLACENTA PREVIA

Placenta previa, which occurs in approximately 1 in 200 to 250 pregnancies, is a condition in which the placenta is positioned abnormally in the uterus in such a way that it covers the cervical opening. Often placenta previa is detected during a routine ultrasound. In other cases, women begin bleeding painlessly in the last trimester of pregnancy. Most women with placenta previa have their first bleeding after their thirtieth week. Many studies have been done about the causes of placenta previa. Some say that it is due to previous uterine surgery, while others say it is due to

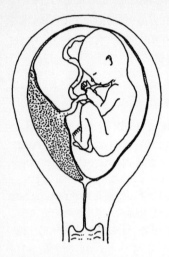 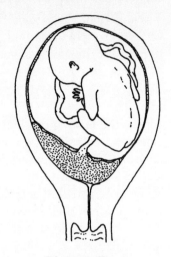

Partial Placentia Previa   **Placentia Previa**

advanced age, a history of many pregnancies, inadequate uterine lining, or congenital abnormalities.

Treatment depends on the severity of your condition but most often includes bed rest to prevent early delivery. Sometimes women are able to rest at home; in other cases hospitalization may be recommended. You will be advised to avoid sexual intercourse, douching, and straining to pass a stool. Stool softeners may be prescribed. A repeat ultrasound will be done later in pregnancy in order to monitor the status of the placenta. Sometimes placenta previa found in an early ultrasound may not persist as the pregnancy progresses.

If you are prior to term, lung maturity tests (see chapter 7) may be done in the event of possible preterm labor. A cesarean is often the delivery of choice.

PROLAPSED UMBILICAL CORD

In this situation, your baby's umbilical cord descends through your cervix into the vagina. A prolapsed umbilical cord has been associated with breech positions and with women who prematurely rupture their membranes. This is an emergency situation because if the fetus's umbilical cord is pinched, the fetus will not receive adequate oxygen.

It will be difficult for you to know if you have a prolapsed umbilical cord. It may be detected by your physician after your membranes have ruptured. Treatment involves an emergency cesarean delivery. In the meantime, you may be told to lie down and get into a knee-to-chest position to relieve some of the pressure on the cord, or you may be told to elevate your hips above your shoulders by lying down and placing a pillow underneath your hips.

INTRAUTERINE GROWTH RETARDATION (IUGR)

IUGR pertains to those infants whose gestational size is 10 percent less than what it should be or under the tenth percentile. This is also known as small size for gestational age (SGA), fetal malnutrition, or dysmaturity. A baby that is small for its age often has a small placenta.

There are many reasons why some babies don't grow as well and as quickly as others. Some of these are chromosomal abnormalities, multiple gestation (and so less room inside the uterus for the baby to grow), poor maternal weight gain, maternal hypertension, infection of the mother, smoking, and alcohol usage. Many of the causes of IUGR are preventable.

IUGR occurs in approximately 5 to 10 percent of all pregnancies, and these babies are at great risk during the first few weeks of life. Ultrasound has helped diagnose IUGR early. Resting on one's side has been recommended to increase blood flow to the placenta.

Treatment for IUGR varies. Repeated ultrasounds are usually done to monitor the baby's status. Other tests such as biophysical profiles and nonstress tests may also be done (see chapter 7). IUGR babies are usually delivered before the thirty-sixth week by cesarean in order to avoid the chance of death, which may occur between the thirty-sixth and fortieth week. The exact timing of the cesarean delivery is highly individual.

PREMATURE RUPTURE OF MEMBRANES (PROM)

PROM is the rupture of the amniotic sac around the fetus before labor begins. It occurs in approximately 10 to 20 percent of all pregnancies. Approximately 20 percent of cases occur before the thirty-sixth week. The exact cause of PROM is unknown; many authorities say that it is usually caused by a uterine infection. Other, less common possible causes include trauma, incompetent cervix, multiple pregnancies, multiple amniocentesis, too much amniotic fluid (polyhydramnios), abruptio placenta, genetic abnormality, poor hygiene, smoking, and inadequate nutrition.

If your membranes rupture prematurely, you will feel a sudden gush of fluid from your vagina. Slow leaks also occur, in which a small amount of liquid leaks from the vagina and is sometimes confused with urine. If this happens to you, you should immediately go to the hospital, because once the sac has been broken there is a greater risk of infection.

Treatment depends upon your stage of pregnancy. For the most part, the management of PROM is highly controversial and often a matter of preference. Today, physicians are somewhat more conservative and many tend to opt for a "wait and see" approach, especially if the woman is less than thirty-six weeks pregnant. If your membranes rupture, labor almost always begins within twenty-four hours. If labor does not occur within twenty-four hours and there are no strong, rhythmic contractions, then labor will be induced in order to prevent infection both of the membranes and in the newborn. Some physicians may choose to wait longer than twenty-four hours.

POSTTERM OR PROLONGED PREGNANCY

Postterm pregnancies or prolonged pregnancies are those that continue past your EDD (expected due date or date of delivery) or EDC (expected date of confinement). Most pregnancies are maintained for thirty-eight to forty-two weeks. However, between 8 and 11 percent of all pregnancies continue longer. Often this is due to the wrong estimated date of conception, when a woman has kept a poor record of her last menstrual cycle. A due date is calculated on the basis of the first day of the last menstrual cycle, and if a woman does not recall the date, the chance of error is larger and the physician must depend upon ultrasound reports to determine the correct fetal age. Despite these indicators, you should understand that your delivery may occur anywhere from two weeks before to two weeks after your expected date of delivery.

Some women are at greater risk for developing a postterm pregnancy; these include women pregnant for the first time, diabetics, those over the age of thirty-five, and those with a history of threatened miscarriage or of a previous prolonged pregnancy.

In many cases, carrying the baby a bit longer will have minimal consequences. However, in other cases it may be associated with placental tears, lack of oxygen supply for the fetus, a large baby, growth retardation, meconium in the amniotic fluid (which indicates distress), or death. The most difficult part of prolonged pregnancies is the emotional aspect. Some women feel as if their pregnancy will never end and they will never get to hold their precious little bundle. It is normal for postterm mothers to feel frustrated and to feel as if they have lost control over their pregnancy.

Ultrasound, oxytocin challenge test, nonstress test, tests of amniotic fluid (for amount and quality), and fetal breathing movement tests will be done to ensure fetal well-being. If the fetus is normal and your cervix is ripe, your physician may choose to induce labor. If your cervix is not soft or you have passed two to three weeks of your EDD, then a cesarean may be considered. In some instances, the cervix may be primed with prostin gel.

If you are past forty weeks, you should be particularly aware of fetal movements and phone your physician immediately if you notice any change. If you have lost more than three pounds in a week, you should also alert your physician. Other indicators for immediate delivery include hypertension, preeclampsia, and any test indicating a fetal problem.

POSTMATURITY

Postmaturity refers to a more serious condition in which the baby's health declines as a result of the delayed birth. The placenta may shrink and the amount of amniotic fluid decrease. When this happens, the baby becomes inadequately nourished and will show signs of distress. A cesarean delivery is necessary.

ECTOPIC PREGNANCY

This type of pregnancy is one in which the egg implants itself outside the uterine wall. About 98 percent of ectopic pregnancies

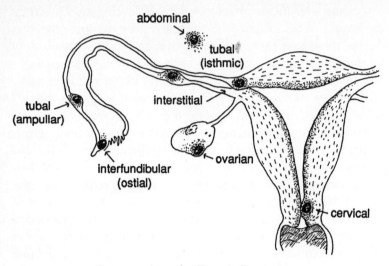

Common Sites for Ectopic Pregnancy

occur in the fallopian tube, although other potential sites include the ovary, the cervix, or the abdominal cavity. Any previous injury or obstruction to the fallopian tube may have resulted in scarring that could affect the egg's journey to the uterus for implantation.

The incidence of ectopic pregnancies has risen over the years and, according to the *New England Journal of Medicine* (1997), approximately one hundred thousand cases are reported each year. Despite this increase, mortality rates have decreased dramatically because of new diagnostic medical and surgical techniques, and women who have had an ectopic pregnancy have a good chance of having a successful pregnancy in the future. The risk factors for developing ectopic pregnancies include the following:

O A history of pelvic inflammatory disease (PID)

O Endometriosis

O A history of tubal adhesions

O Previous surgery to the fallopian tubes or pelvic cavity

O Previous ectopic pregnancy

O DES exposure

Early diagnosis of an ectopic pregnancy is critical for saving the woman's life and safeguarding her future ability to bear children. Some early telltale signs include a missed period, abdominal pain (mild at first, then becoming severe), vaginal bleeding, fainting, and a mass in your abdomen. The first sign will probably be pain in your lower abdomen. Some women have a dull, aching pain, while others may experience excruciating pain. One woman said that she had such intense pain she thought her appendix had ruptured.

If you have any of these symptoms, you should call your physician. He or she will perform an examination that will probably feel a bit uncomfortable. Blood tests and an ultrasound will also be done to verify you are pregnant. Next, a laparoscopy will be done so that your abdominal and pelvic area may be examined. If an ectopic pregnancy is diagnosed, there are a number of treatments available, depending on your status.

Conservative medical treatment may include administering methotrexate, an anticancer medication that dissolves placental and embryonic tissue and eliminates the risk of surgical damage to the fallopian tubes and subsequent infertility. This treatment, however, is not widely used. Its main advantage is that it may be used prior to bleeding from ectopic pregnancy.

Some women may not require any medication, as their ectopic pregnancy may be reabsorbed by their body. In other cases microsurgery may be done to remove the products of conception and to preserve the fallopian tube.

If you are having excruciating pain, your tube may have ruptured, in which case immediate surgery will be necessary to remove the tubal pregnancy and sometimes the affected fallopian tube as well. Awaiting the surgery may be very uncomfortable for you. It is best that you remain calm and stay in a comfortable position. Sitting or standing usually intensifies the discomfort in the rectal area, and for some women lying down intensifies shoulder pain, especially if there was bleeding in the abdomen as a result of the rupture.

Facing surgery for ectopic pregnancy is difficult. You will be facing not only the normal fear of the surgical procedure, but the possible outcome of the loss of fertility. It is not all dismal, however. Ectopic surgery may decrease your chances of being able to conceive again, but it does not eliminate the possibility of a future pregnancy. In all probability you will experience all the anger and concerns that accompany loss. Speaking with other women who have been through a similar experience may help you cope.

HYDATIFORM MOLE

A hydatiform mole is an abnormal development of the placenta that results in a benign or malignant tumor. It is a rare condition in which a developing pregnancy degenerates and the placental tissue forms a grape-like mass called a hydatiform mole. It occurs in about one in fifteen hundred pregnancies in the United States and is eight times more common in East Asia. It is also more common in women under twenty and over forty. The causes are unknown, although it has been associated with nutritional deficiency, chromosomal abnormalities, and hormonal imbalance.

The symptoms include extreme nausea, bleeding, an unusually large uterus for the time in pregnancy, signs of preeclampsia, and the absence of fetal heart sounds. It is usually suspected late in the first trimester or early in the second trimester.

The treatment options include vacuum aspiration, as done for abortion, oxytocin or prostaglandin induction to expel the contents of the uterus or, more rarely, hysterectomy. In some cases, women who have hydatiform mole are predisposed to developing uterine cancer. If your childbearing years are nearing an end, hysterectomy may be recommended. If cancer is present, chemotherapy will be initiated. If uterine cancer is diagnosed early enough, chemotherapy is very effective, and the woman may be able to become pregnant at a later date.

The loss that a woman feels following this operation may be similar to that of a miscarriage, since she thought she was having a baby up until the diagnosis was made. Some women may have odd feelings, such as feeling like a "freak" or feeling less feminine and desirable. It is important that you continue to look after yourself and be good to yourself.

COPING WITH HIGH-RISK PREGNANCY

Whatever problem you have that makes you a candidate for high-risk pregnancy, the days ahead will not be easy. At times, you may feel scared and uncertain. One tip is to take one day at a time and to think of the stress of the situation as an opportunity for growth. There are many stages that high-risk mothers pass through that help them cope with their situation. First, you need to accept your pregnancy and the risks that it involves. Sometimes this is difficult, and women may find themselves denying that there is any problem. Chances are that the sooner you accept your high-risk pregnancy, the easier it will be for you to follow your physician's recommendations. Some women have to give up certain activities or jobs in order to safely carry their baby. Having to take a leave of absence from work may be very stressful. Speaking with your employer about returning may help to relieve some pressure. If this is uncomfortable for you, it may be a good idea to speak with the social-service department of your hospital, which may be able to serve as a liaison between you and your employer. In some instances, you may also be eligible for disability insurance benefits. Seeking support from professionals, relatives, and friends is also very important.

It is common to feel shocked when you are first told about your high-risk pregnancy. You may feel a sense of disbelief and may not actually hear the details of your physician's explanation. It is important to ask any questions that come to mind and to ask for further explanations at a later date. Keep a notepad in your purse, because concerns may come to you at the most unusual times!

It is normal to ask yourself "Why me?" when faced with a problem pregnancy. Seeking the attention of specialists to find solutions to your problems is more productive than mulling over why it has happened to you. Understanding the reason for your problem will help you to cope with it. If your problem pregnancy may result in a child with disabilities, now is your chance to prepare for life after the birth. There are many excellent organizations that can help you (see Appendix C).

High-risk pregnancies sometimes result in the death of a child. Understandably, couples facing a high-risk pregnancy always have this in the back of their minds. Feelings of guilt are normal but rarely justified. Couples need to remind themselves that everything was done in the baby-to-be's best interest and that medical science cannot perform miracles. Having the support of those around her is very important to a woman enduring a high-risk pregnancy. Having a supportive and understanding husband and family, in addition to a supportive and caring physician, is very important.

Feelings of hopelessness, discouragement, anxiety, and depression are all normal for the high-risk mother. It is natural to be bothered by women who are having "normal" pregnancies. It is not unusual to be envious of other mothers-to-be who can just get into their car and drive to the shopping center. High-risk mothers are often on edge. They learn to take one day at a time. This is what is unique about high-risk pregnancies. They are so dynamic. What may be okay today may not be okay tomorrow. For women in this situation, there is no reason to feel guilty. If you have questions about what is happening or what will happen, the best thing to do is ask your physician. Very often you will imagine your predicament to be much worse than it really is.

Dr. Robert Knuppel, an OB/GYN whose practice is primarily devoted to high-risk pregnancies, says that most of his high-risk patients have previously had complications and that "most women have been traumatized and sensitized." It is important to understand that most often you did nothing to cause your problem and that if you have any questions, you should ask them. Most professionals will give you the answers you want to hear, but none will guarantee that "everything will be all right"—so try not to expect them to tell you that. The hours, days, and months may seem endless, but remember that it is not forever and that, after all, you are in bed not because you are sick but because you are awaiting one of life's happiest moments—bringing a child into the world!

HELPFUL PUBLICATIONS

Diabetes and Pregnancy
HIV Testing and Pregnancy
American College of Obstetricians and Gynecologists
ACOG Distribution Center
P.O. Box 4500
Kearneysville, WV 25430-4500

The Bed Rest Survival Guide
    by Barbara Edelston Peterson and Hallie Beachum
Avon Books
1350 Avenue of the Americas
New York, NY 10019
(800) 223-0690

Diabetes in Pregnancy
HIV and AIDS in Pregnancy
The March of Dimes Foundation
Community Services Department
1275 Mamaroneck Avenue
White Plains, NY 10605

Chapter 6

─────────── ◯ ───────────

Sexuality and Nutrition
for Pregnant Women

Humans are different from other species in that our desire for sexual contact continues during pregnancy. In fact, we are the only species that copulates during pregnancy. Our sexual relations are not reserved only for the purpose of making children but are also our way of expressing love. Sexuality, therefore, refers not only to the sexual act but also to how we feel about ourselves. It is normal for pregnancy to cause changing attitudes toward sexuality in both the mother- and the father-to-be. Couples need to be open about their sexual needs and concerns with each other and with their caregivers.

SEXUAL DESIRE

Changes in the desire for sexual contact are common during pregnancy and can be a result of many different factors—physiological and emotional well-being, cultural background, and attitudes toward pregnancy itself. Some women feel they are more attractive during pregnancy, while others are not at all overjoyed by their appearance. Some women take special care to always look and feel good throughout their pregnancy. Research has shown that women tend to experience a decrease in sexual desire in the first trimester, an increase in the second trimester, and a decline again in the third trimester. Although these changes may be hormonal, it is clear that the normal complaints of early pregnancy, such as nausea and fatigue, can strongly affect sexual desire. Toward the end of pregnancy, when a woman has substantially increased in size, sex may not be as comfortable or as exciting. In addition, the latter part of pregnancy is accompanied by feelings that are more strongly maternal than romantic. Fluctuations in sexual desire are normal during pregnancy, and therefore you should not be overly concerned if you alternate between feeling oversexed and undersexed.

Some couples, especially high-risk ones, may be afraid of hurting the fetus during sexual relations and therefore restrain or avoid intimacy. Many high-risk mothers are reluctant to ask their obstetricians about sexual activity and prefer the "better safe than sorry" approach.

Much of the literature focuses on the female sexual response during pregnancy. However, we must not forget the feelings of the male partner. The father-to-be also undergoes significant changes associated with pregnancy, and, although not physiologically based, these emotional issues may dramatically affect his sexual needs and desires. The new role of fatherhood brings with it many fears and uncertainties. The woman's bodily changes, such as increased breast size, swollen vagina, and protruding abdomen, may elicit varying responses in her partner. The man may feel unsure about sexual relations during pregnancy and may have difficulty expressing this fear. Feeling afraid is common among men and may be one reason for decreased sexual relations among some couples. If relations are resumed, the man may be unable to maintain an erection or to achieve orgasm because of the fear of injuring the unborn child. Other men may find the pregnant woman very attractive and feel an increase in sexual desire.

SAFETY OF SEX

Sexual contact is an intimacy between two people. The type of intimacy depends upon the individuals. While some couples are quite content cuddling and touching, the vast majority equate intimacy with the act of sexual intercourse.

It is important for you and your partner to voice your concerns about your sexual activity during pregnancy, because talking about it often relieves a great deal of tension. If you have any anxiety about the safety of sexual relations, you should discuss it with your physician. If you are advised to refrain from intercourse and/or orgasm, you can find alternative ways to express your love for each other.

For those who choose alternatives to sexual intercourse during pregnancy, it is important to know that there may be some risks. For example, because masturbation in women often provides a more intense orgasm than intercourse, your physician may recommend that you refrain from it. Those engaging in oral sex should note that air blown into the vagina may create the risk of an air embolism. This act should be carried out with extreme caution during pregnancy.

More often than not, in normal pregnancies there is no evidence of orgasm or sexual intercourse adversely affecting the fetus or triggering bleeding, miscarriage, or preterm labor. If you are having a high-risk pregnancy you should ask your caregiver if intercourse and/or orgasm is recommended. It is very common to experience some brief abdominal cramping following intercourse. If this continues or gets worse over a one-hour period, contact your physician, since it may be possible that your cervix is dilating. In general, intercourse is not advised during three specific times: if there is bleeding during pregnancy, for the first four weeks following vaginal childbirth, and for six weeks following cesarean birth.

For the most part, sexual intercourse during pregnancy is both appropriate and healthy for both partners. There are some positions that tend to be more safe than others for the pregnant woman and a few examples are illustrated below. These are taken from the pamphlet *Some Things About Sex and Pregnancy* by Ann Hager, R.N.

Following are some situations in which you may be advised to refrain from intercourse.

Vaginal Bleeding

Whether bleeding is during the first, second, or third trimester, intercourse is not recommended. Bleeding during the early months can be indicative of impending miscarriage; if the miscarriage is due to a blighted ovum (an egg that does not develop properly), intercourse will not affect its outcome. Bleeding in the

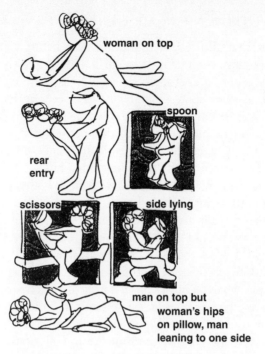

woman on top

spoon

rear
entry

scissors

side lying

man on top but
woman's hips
on pillow, man
leaning to one side

Alternative Positions for High-Risk Couples

second and third trimesters may be due to uterine abnormalities
or problems with the placenta, such as placenta previa and abruptio placenta. Your physician will probably recommend that you
refrain from intercourse to prevent any problems.

Rupture of Membranes

Intercourse is not recommended once your membranes have ruptured, because it may result in a serious uterine infection. And if
you ever feel a gush of fluid from your vagina, you should refrain
from intercourse and immediately phone your physician.

Other Problems

Uterine fibroids, congenital uterine abnormalities, and incompetent cervix are other situations in which your physician may
advise you to refrain from sexual intercourse.

NUTRITION FOR A HEALTHY PREGNANCY

Good maternal nutrition should begin even before you are pregnant. If you have been taking the Pill, you have already been taking special care. After stopping the Pill, it is recommended that you give your body approximately one to three months to replenish itself. It is recommended that you take a vitamin B complex and folic acid supplement during this period. It is also recommended that you continue taking folic acid during the first months of pregnancy to help prevent spina bifida.

During pregnancy—probably more than any other time in your life—you need to eat well. Although *you* may not be sensitive to dietary changes, your baby is, and it may be at risk for developing problems if you are not careful. Pregnancy is not a time for dieting. Dieting will deprive the fetus of the valuable nutritional support that it needs to grow. Severe dieting can have serious consequences. For example, when fat breaks down during dieting, toxic substances called ketone bodies are released. These can harm the fetus.

Eating a well-balanced diet with foods from all of the four food groups is the basis of good nutrition. Caloric requirements increase during pregnancy as the body strives to meet the needs of two persons. Women who are close to their ideal body weight do not need any additional calories during the first trimester. It is usually recommended that, beginning in the second trimester, pregnant women increase their daily caloric intake by 300 to 500 calories. If you are exercising less or are on bed rest, you will need to adjust your caloric intake accordingly.

In addition to the extra calories, a pregnant woman's diet must provide certain nutrients to ensure proper fetal growth and development. These are indicated in the chart on the facing page.

Weight Gain

During the first three months of pregnancy, a woman will normally gain between two and three pounds. From the beginning of the fourth month and until term, a steady gain of about one pound per week is desirable, although a spurt of two pounds is not unusual. There should be a steady weight increase.

Diet Guidelines for a Healthy Pregnancy

Nutrients	Food Group	Food Type	Daily Servings
Protein and Iron	Meat	meats, fish, poultry, eggs, nuts, legumes, cereals, pasta	four 3-oz servings
Calcium	Milk	milk, yogurt, cheese	four 8-oz servings or 1 oz of cheese
Vitamins A and C	Fruits and Vegetables	citrus fruits, leafy green vegetables, potatoes, unsweetened juices, vegetable juices	five servings, 1 cup raw, ½ cup cooked
B Vitamins	Bread	whole-grain bread, fortified cereals, pasta, rice	four to six servings
Fluids		water	six to eight servings

Certain changes in weight may indicate a problem. For example, a sudden weight gain in the second half of pregnancy accompanied by elevated blood pressure may be a warning sign of preeclampsia. Loss of weight or a failure to gain weight in the latter part of pregnancy is also a sign of a potential complication. There is usually a small weight loss when labor is imminent. This is due to a decrease in fluid retention caused by a drop in progesterone, which usually promotes fluid retention.

Women who start off thin are usually expected to gain between twenty-eight and thirty-six pounds. Overweight women should gain between sixteen and twenty-four pounds in order to avoid problems and labor difficulties.

Approximate Weight Gain in Pregnancy

fetus	7.5 pounds
placenta	1.5
amniotic fluid	2.0
uterus	2.5
breasts	1.0–3.0
extra blood	4.0
body fluids	2.0
maternal store	4.0–8.0
TOTAL	24.5–30.5 pounds

NUTRIENT SUPPLEMENTATION

Nutrition in pregnancy is a delicate balance of taking the correct nutrients while maintaining a reasonable caloric intake. Although a well-balanced diet will provide all the required nutrients, there are certain nutrient supplements that may be required under supervision during pregnancy, including iron, calcium, vitamin D, and folic acid.

Iron A daily iron supplement providing 30 to 60 mg of iron will usually be prescribed. Iron supplements, however, should be taken under supervision.

There are a number of women who are at risk for iron deficiency, including those who become pregnant with low iron stores, those carrying twins, those who were underweight or malnourished when they became pregnant, adolescents, those with closely spaced pregnancies, those with a history of fertility problems, and those who have had previous gastric surgery. Iron-rich foods, in combination with an iron supplement, may be recommended.

Iron is best absorbed on an empty stomach, but it may cause gastrointestinal discomfort. It is often recommended that iron supplements be taken with a meal containing vitamin C and/or meats and poultry, which enhance iron absorption in the body. Red meats are the source of iron, which is best absorbed by the body. Milk, tea, coffee, cola, and other caffeine-containing beverages tend to reduce iron absorption and should be avoided at meals, especially when iron-rich foods are served.

A word of caution: vitamin supplements fortified with iron often cause constipation. Instead of taking laxatives during pregnancy, it is advised that you eat foods with bulk and fiber, drink prune juice, and increase your daily water consumption. Some dieticians recommend drinking a cup of hot water on an empty stomach first thing in the morning to alleviate constipation. Also, do not be alarmed if your stool turns black—this is caused by the extra iron in your system. The iron in prenatal supplements may also cause a red and itchy rash over the torso. In this case, it is best to stop the vitamin supplement for a few days. Speak to your physician about another iron source.

Although prenatal blood tests include a blood count to determine your hemoglobin, you may at a later date find you are constantly overtired. You should mention this to your nutritionist or physician, who will recheck your iron level at twenty-eight weeks. If you are a vegetarian or prefer not to eat too much meat, there are many other sources. Remember that these are best absorbed when eaten with acidic foods.

Sources of Iron

- O Red meat

- O Egg yolk

- O Almonds

- O Peaches, apricots, prunes, raisins

- O Beans

- O Kidneys

- O Bran (in moderation)

- O Liver

- O Oatmeal

- O Oysters

- O Fortified breads and cereals

Calcium A total of 1,200 mg of calcium daily is recommended during pregnancy. Pregnant adolescents should add an additional 400 mg daily. Calcium is needed during pregnancy for developing the bones and teeth of the fetus, and it is most needed in the second and third trimesters of pregnancy, when bone formation occurs. Women needing calcium supplementation are those with lactose intolerance or milk allergies, or those who simply do not like drinking milk. Those who have lactose intolerance will be advised on the use of the enzymes that facilitate its digestion. Sometimes those with lactose intolerance find it easier to digest hard cheeses, unprocessed cheeses (e.g., cheddar, Swiss), yogurt, and canned fish with bones. Vegetarians who use soy milk should know that this contains half the calcium of cow's milk, and therefore the quantity consumed should be doubled. Vegetables such as broccoli, spinach, and mustard greens also supply calcium, though calcium from vegetable sources is less easily absorbed by the body.

Vitamin D Vitamin D is essential for calcium's absorption in the body. It also plays a role in mineralizing the baby's skeletal system. Today, milk and margarine are fortified with vitamin D. However, those at most risk for vitamin D deficiency are vegetarians, those who dislike milk, and those taking anticonvulsants. Exposure to sunlight also provides vitamin D, but if you are pregnant during the winter months, this exposure is often limited and you may be advised to take a vitamin supplement or to increase your dietary intake of this vitamin. Some dietary fiber tends to inhibit lactose absorption, while some sugars increase its absorption.

Folic Acid Folic acid is one of the vitamin B-complex group and is important for cell division and blood formation. It may help prevent spina bifida and related birth defects that occur during the third week of gestation. It is very important during pregnancy because of the increased number of cells being produced by the mother: a pregnant woman will need about three to four times more folic acid than the nonpregnant woman. The recommended dosage is about 400 mg. Folic acid is destroyed when cooked at high temperatures, so you should limit microwave cooking, as it destroys more folic acid than conventional cooking methods. When cooking vegetables it is a good idea to use smaller amounts of water, as water will dilute the folic acid present in the vegetables. In addition, there is considerable loss of this vitamin due to oxidation when food has been stored for more than a few days, making it difficult to obtain in food sources. Women at greatest risk of developing folic acid deficiency are those with multiple pregnancies, absorption problems, or anemia, and those on anticonvulsant and steroid medications (such as betamethasone, prescribed for fetal lung maturity). To help reduce the risk, women should take folic acid two months before conception and at least during the first month of pregnancy.

Sources of Folic Acid

○ Meat

○ Asparagus

○ Green leafy vegetables (spinach, romaine lettuce)

○ Kidney

○ Lima beans

○ Liver

○ Eggs

○ Nuts

○ Yeast

○ Fish

Sodium The volume of water in a woman's body increases when she is pregnant. As a result, she needs to increase the total amount of body sodium in proportion to her caloric intake to maintain her body's chemical balance. In the past, salt was not recommended for pregnant women. Theories have changed, however, and the current belief is that you should salt your foods to taste. Processed foods have large amounts of salt and should be used in moderation.

Protein Protein is essential for building fetal tissues. It provides the body with energy and is needed for the manufacture of hormones, antibodies, enzymes, and tissues. For her protein to be used by the fetal tissues, the mother must consume adequate amounts of calories to meet the daily energy requirement of both mother and child. A pregnant woman should increase her protein intake to an average of 70 to 90 g daily. Most protein-containing foods are also good sources of vitamins and minerals. Vegetarians can add protein to their diet by combining grains with beans or nuts, and combining any of these with dairy products on the same day. They may also need to supplement their diet with vitamins or to use soy protein in cooking. Yogurt is an excellent source of protein and also contains vitamins A and D, as well as many B-complex vitamins.

Fluids Water is important because it transports vital nutrients from one part of the body to another. It is also a very necessary part of chemical reactions, such as the breaking down of complex nutrients into smaller units. Our bodies are constantly losing water, through sweating, urinating, and breathing. We also lose water through vomiting and diarrhea.

Pregnant women need to drink more fluids. In addition to the milk requirement, it is important for them to drink at least six glasses of water daily. Recent studies show that caffeine can increase the risk of miscarriage. Women should limit their caffeine intake to one product per day.

Vitamin Supplementation

Vitamin supplementation during pregnancy is controversial. Some caregivers recommend it in special cases, while others recommend it for all their patients. Many caregivers recommend vitamin and mineral supplements even prior to conception. Whenever possible, nutritional deficiencies should be corrected by food rather than by supplementation. Discuss this carefully with your physician, as too much of some nutrients, such as vitamin A, may have the potential to cause serious birth defects.

Tips on Prenatal Vitamins

1. Take the prescribed dose (usually one per day). Do not take megavitamins or begin any special vitamin program without medical supervision. Some nutrients may cause birth defects.

2. If you find that taking your prenatal vitamin nauseates you, or if you feel like regurgitating it, take it with some food. If this doesn't help, tell your physician. He or she may recommend not taking it for a week or so.

3. Keep vitamins and other medications out of the reach of small children. In an attempt to "copy mommy," a toddler may think that pills are like candy. Iron pills can kill.

NUTRITION GUIDELINES FOR SPECIAL SITUATIONS

For the high-risk mother, nutrition guidelines may be a bit challenging. Following is a summary of nutritional guidelines for some of the special situations that a high-risk mother may face. These are only suggestions, and you should consult your physician before trying anything discussed here.

Anemia

Anemia is caused by a lowered hemoglobin level or a decrease in the number of red blood cells. Since hemoglobin carries your body's oxygen concentration in the blood, it is important that its level be kept adequate. During pregnancy, your blood volume increases by 33 percent, which means that there are more red blood cells with less hemoglobin. As a result, many health care professionals believe that vitamin supplements fortified with iron are necessary to meet this additional requirement.

There are various types of anemia, but iron-deficiency anemia is the one most commonly seen in pregnancy. Vitamin supplements and food sources such as red meat, liver, leafy green vegetables, apples, apricots, bananas, egg yolks, prunes, raisins, squash, and whole grains, taken with vitamin C, help to increase iron absorption.

If left untreated, anemia has risks for the unborn child, as it jeopardizes the baby's supply of oxygen and essential nutrients. It can affect the baby's growth and consequently its birth size. If the anemia is severe, stillbirth is possible.

A lack of folic acid (a vitamin needed for red blood cell division) and vitamin B-12 may cause problems similar to those of iron deficiency. Without folic acid, red blood cells do not divide; they become enlarged and fewer in number, causing folic acid anemia.

Toxemias and Hypertension

Preventing malnutrition in the pregnant woman has long been correlated with preventing toxemia of pregnancy. Proper nutrition and an increased protein intake when you have toxemia can help to prevent more serious complications of the illness.

Adequate protein in the diet is important for the metabolism, especially to maintain adequate fluid, electrolyte balance, and fat transport. Sodium or salt restriction is sometimes recommended in toxemia to minimize water retention and swelling.

Certain vitamins are of particular importance to the toxemic mother. Vitamins such as A, C, D, and B-complex are related to protein and energy metabolism. Studies have shown that placentas of toxemic women have about one-third the normal amount of vitamin B-6.

Heart Disease

The nutritional alterations necessary for cardiac disease are similar to those for toxemia. Under supervision, you should maintain an appropriate weight and restrict sodium to 2 to 3 g per day. Salty foods such as smoked meats, pickles, relishes, and condiments should all be avoided. You should never be on a restrictive diet without the advice of your physician. Fad diets or "crash" diets can be downright dangerous. Proper weight control means avoiding empty caloric foods and excessive quantities of food.

Multiple Pregnancy

There are conflicting opinions about whether the mother's nutritional requirements actually double or quadruple with a multiple pregnancy. The only way to assess adequate nutrition is by blood tests, fetal growth, and weight gain. Small and frequent meals may help the woman to consume larger amounts of food. Vitamin supplementation may be recommended. It is important to have adequate prenatal care and perhaps to be monitored by a dietician if you have any questions.

Diabetes

Diet and/or insulin control of diabetes will need to be carefully monitored during pregnancy. Women who were diabetic prior to pregnancy have the highest chance of problems and need to be followed very closely. The fetus has the greatest chance of developing birth defects during the first five to eight weeks of pregnancy, before most women know they are pregnant. Whether you had diabetes prior to pregnancy or develop gestational diabetes, a dietician should plan your diet.

He or she will carefully consider the amount of energy you expend during a day and will weigh this against your nutritional requirements and those of your baby. If you are diabetic and for some other reason must be on bed rest, this will also be taken into consideration, and your caloric intake will need to be slightly lower than that of an active nonpregnant woman, without depriving your baby.

Complex carbohydrates, such as starches (whole-grain bread, pasta, cereals, corn, peas, beans) and vegetables, will be recommended and should make up 50 to 55 percent of your diet. Recent research shows that juices are absorbed very fast. The absorption rate also depends upon the other foods being eaten at the same time.

Protein is also very important in diabetes, and 20 to 22 percent of your total caloric intake should be from protein.

In addition to its benefits to the intestinal tract, fiber has been identified as a useful food in controlling diabetes, as it influences the body's general metabolism. If you are not used to eating high-fiber foods, you should add fiber to your diet slowly. Especially if you are having a high-risk pregnancy with a risk of preterm labor, you should check with your physician before eating high-fiber foods. Sudden usage in large amounts can cause cramps and could stimulate uterine contractions.

Sources of Fiber

○ Raw vegetables

○ Raw fruits

O Whole-grain cereals

O Legumes

O Nuts

O Bran (in moderation)

O Prunes

Three meals a day with midmorning, midafternoon, and evening snacks will also be recommended. If you are on insulin it is very important to have regular and consistent meals. You may be taught to test your own blood sugar level before and after meals. Certain medications, such as Ritodrine, which prevents preterm labor, and steroids such as cortisone have the tendency to temporarily raise the blood-sugar level, which makes women using them more prone to diabetes in pregnancy if they have some of the other risk factors mentioned earlier. These women should be even more careful to restrict their total caloric intake. Ritodrine may also cause nausea and vomiting in some women. You should notify your physician if you have these symptoms so that a special diet can be formulated. Taking smaller and more frequent meals is often recommended.

Birth Interval

The optimal interval between pregnancies has not been established. However, there is a greater incidence of lags in fetal growth and prematurity if the birth interval is less than two years. Certain nutrients may not be adequately replenished within that time. If you have had more than one baby in two years, you should meet with a nutritionist to ensure that you and your baby are getting adequate nourishment. A vitamin supplement may be recommended.

Bed Rest

The nutritional needs of the woman on bed rest are different, because of her diminished activity level. She may find it difficult to maintain good nutritional habits. Some women find their appetite is diminished due to less activity, while others find that they are bored and that eating is a perfect time-filler. Often the woman is unable to choose and prepare her favorite foods and loses her appetite. Being on bed rest may predispose some women to feelings of heartburn, which can further diminish their appetite.

Avoiding empty-calorie foods such as cakes, cookies, and candies is important for all pregnant women, but especially for the woman on bed rest. When you eat anything, especially sweets, it stimulates the pancreas to secrete insulin to help metabolize the sugar and other ingredients. About one hour later the blood glucose level falls rapidly, and the fetus also experiences this rapid shift. A relatively constant blood-sugar level is much better for the development of the fetus. This is not to say that sweets are not permitted at all, but they should be taken in small amounts and with other high-protein foods.

Chapter 7

———————O———————

Tests, Tests, Tests

Tests during pregnancy are inevitable. They answer many questions and help to provide a sense of security about what is going on. Medical testing today is quite a bit more sophisticated than it was years ago. Women know a lot about their pregnancies, and they know much more than they used to about what to expect.

The first time you meet with your physician, you will be asked various questions about your past and present health, for example, When was your first menstrual period? What is the duration of your period? How heavy is the flow? How long is your cycle? Were you ever pregnant before? Did you ever have any abortions? Miscarriages? Do you have any health problems? Are you taking any medications? Have you ever had urinary or vaginal infections? You may be asked questions about your mother's history, since many female characteristics are inherited.

The information you provide gives a baseline history that will subsequently help in planning your prenatal care. For example, if there is a family history of genetic disorders, such as hemophilia, Downs syndrome, or birth defects, your physician may recommend certain genetic-screening tests. If you have had uterine fibroids (benign tumors on the wall of the uterus), an ultrasound may be recommended to detect their presence, size, and growth rate. Tests may be done at various times during your pregnancy to assist the physician in detecting any high-risk problems before they arise.

PREGNANCY TESTS

Whether you are a potential high-risk mother or not, the first step is to have a pregnancy test to ensure that you are pregnant. Over the years there have been many types of pregnancy tests, some more accurate than others. The accuracy of the results depends upon the test's sensitivity.

Pregnancy tests, whether blood or urine tests, check for the presence of human chorionic gonadotropin (hCG), a hormone produced by the placenta shortly after conception. hCG is detectable eight to ten days after conception. A positive test, in conjunction with other signs, will help confirm your pregnancy.

Some Early Signs of Pregnancy

○ Missed period

○ Breast fullness

○ Darkened areola

○ Aching in lower abdomen

○ Increased vaginal secretions

○ Increased urinary frequency

○ Nausea/vomiting

○ Fatigue

○ Positive pregnancy test

Years ago, women would go to their physician if they suspected they were pregnant. Today, many women go to the nearest store and buy a home test. Others may choose to go to the health department, a midwife's office, or, in some areas, local pharmacies that will perform a urine test on a first-in-the-morning urine specimen. Although the pharmaceutical industry is beginning to meet the needs of today's busy woman by improving on the home pregnancy test, these home-based tests are generally not as accurate as the ones done in the pharmacy or hospital.

Home tests detect pregnancy by measuring the amount of hCG in your urine. hCG causes menstruation to stop, and these tests may be done from the first to the third day after a missed period onward.

It is important to check the expiration date on the kit prior to performing any tests. Be sure to follow the instructions exactly.

To collect your specimen, use a first-in-the-morning urine sample collected in a clean and dry container (sometimes provided). If you are unable to perform the test immediately, the urine should be covered and refrigerated and the test done later on the same day. However, before doing the test, allow the urine to come to room temperature. The urine at the top of the container should be tested.

Most of the tests are done relatively quickly and take from two minutes to one hour. If your urine is cloudy, pink, or red, or has a strong odor, wait a few days to do the test. Talk to your physician or pharmacist if you have any questions.

If you think you are pregnant but the test is negative, count again the number of days since your last period and repeat the test a few days later. There is a chance that not enough hCG has accumulated in your urine to provide a positive result. If your test remains negative and you still do not have a period, consult your physician, as there may be another reason for your missed period.

The earlier you know you are pregnant, the sooner you will be able to take care of yourself and that precious life inside of you. Your physician will be able to detect your pregnancy after your second missed period through other signs, such as your uterus being larger than usual, your breasts being more tender, and the color of your vagina changing to a purplish hue. After your examination, your physician will probably recommend another pregnancy test.

If your physician suspects an ectopic pregnancy, a hydatiform mole, or a threatened miscarriage, he or she may recommend a pregnancy test called a B-hCG blood test. If you fall into any of these categories, your placenta will secrete either too much or too little of the hormone hCG. This test is the most sensitive pregnancy test available today because it is the only one that detects very minute levels of hCG. It is done either by a blood or a urine test; the blood test is often more accurate. Results are usually available anywhere from one to forty-eight hours later.

PRENATAL FOLLOW-UP

Once pregnancy has been confirmed, your prenatal follow-up will begin. The types of tests done from this point on are highly individualized. The following discussion offers some general idea of what to expect; all details should be discussed with your physician.

The First Visit

In most cases, your physician will do a complete physical examination, including a vaginal and breast exam, once your pregnancy is confirmed. If a Pap smear has not been done recently, it will also probably be done at this time. If your examination goes well, you will be told to return in about four to six weeks until the twenty-eighth week, every four weeks thereafter until the thirty-sixth week, and then every one to two weeks until labor begins. If you are having a high-risk pregnancy, these time intervals may be slightly altered.

Testing for gonorrhea, syphilis, chlamydia, and other infections is commonly done early in pregnancy to ensure your baby's safety. These tests are routine; you should not feel that your physician is suspicious of anything in particular.

Due Date

During one of your early prenatal visits, your physician will determine your expected date of delivery (EDD). Knowing the approximate due date is of particular importance in high-risk pregnancies. Should your baby be in distress during your pregnancy, your physician's interventions will depend upon your due date.

Charts are available to give quick answers to your questions, but if you want to know how your EDD was determined, you can figure it out yourself by counting forty weeks or 280 days from the first day of your last period. An even easier way is using Naegele's rule: add seven days to the first day of your last period; subtract three months; add one year. This will be your expected due date. Remember, this is just an estimated date based on women who have menstrual cycles of twenty-eight days. If your cycle is irregular, your ovulation time will be different, as will your due date.

BLOOD AND URINE TESTS

A number of tests may be done to assess your baby's well-being by checking the levels of certain chemicals in your blood or urine.

Years ago, before the widespread use of ultrasound, a wide variety of blood tests were commonplace in high-risk pregnancies.

Blood tests will be done either in your physician's office or in a local hospital or clinic. These initial blood tests will provide the following information:

Blood group and rhesus factor

O Rubella immunity

O Blood count (in case of anemia)

O The presence of blood disorders (e.g., thalessemia, sickle cell disease, hepatitis)

O The presence of AIDS, syphilis, hepatitis B, etc.

You will also be asked to supply a urine sample to be checked for infections. These urine tests are done on a midstream sample, which means that you urinate a little into the toilet, allow some of the remaining urine to go into the specimen cup, and then complete the urination in the toilet. Urine tests will also be performed on each prenatal visit in your physician's office to detect sugar (glucose) or protein in your urine.

Rhesus-Factor Titers

Most people have in their blood a factor called the Rhesus (Rh) factor. These people are considered to be Rh-positive. If you do not have this factor, then you are Rh-negative. There may be a problem of Rh incompatibility if the mother is Rh-negative and the baby is Rh-positive (see chapter 5). Rh-negative mothers are given a series of blood tests (Rh titers) during their pregnancy. If the tests show that the antibodies are increasing, labor may be induced to prevent the fetus's blood from being destroyed.

ULTRASOUND TESTS

An ultrasound is a painless and apparently safe method of scanning your abdomen with high-frequency sound waves to assess your baby's growth and development. These sound waves have a

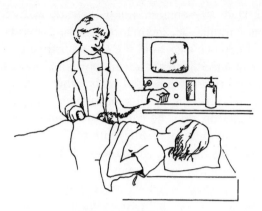

Ultrasound Testing

frequency of approximately twenty thousand vibrations per second. The ultrasound transducer, placed on your abdomen during the examination, emits high-frequency sound waves that pass into the body and are reflected back to the transducer, which also serves as the receiver. The variation in rate and intensity of the sound waves is interpreted electronically to form a picture of the medium through which they pass. In this case, the medium is your abdomen.

Ultrasound scans are known by different names. You might hear them called Doptone, Sonicaid, or Doppler ultrasound.

Uses of Ultrasound Testing

Your physician may recommend that you have an ultrasound around your fourth month. This is done to establish your due date, to scan the fetal organs for abnormalities, and to check the placenta and amniotic fluid surrounding the baby. Most ultrasounds take at least fifteen minutes. Most technicians take longer to ensure that they obtain all the essential information. At present, routine ultrasounds are controversial in "normal" pregnancies. Some physicians do not recommend them at all unless there is a problem, while others advocate one ultrasound early in pregnancy and another at a later date.

Vaginal ultrasounds (sonograms) may be used early in pregnancy if a heartbeat is undetectable or to confirm the date of pregnancy. They are sometimes done as early as five weeks to detect the gestational sac, and in fact, pregnancy may be detected as early as thirty-two days from the last menstrual period. Some physicians claim that with the advent of vaginal sonograms, they are not as surprised as they used to be when a miscarriage or ectopic pregnancy occurs. Ectopic pregnancies detected by vaginal ultrasounds can then be treated by injection of drugs like methotrexate (an anticancer drug) into the gestational sac.

For those with high-risk pregnancies ultrasound may become a frequent experience, since it may help detect potential problems before they occur. What an amazing feeling it is seeing this image on the screen. The baby-to-be finally becomes something tangible rather than an imaginary image. When your baby's image appears on the ultrasound screen, your physician is able to measure its head, leg, and abdomen size—which are all good indicators of growth.

There are many high-risk situations in which ultrasound is done almost routinely. Some of these situations are discussed in the following sections.

Vaginal Bleeding During the First Twenty Weeks As discussed earlier, there are many potential causes of vaginal bleeding, and your physician may have ruled out some of them. One possible cause is an ectopic pregnancy. After a preliminary diagnosis has been made by a physical examination and hCG levels have been tested, an ultrasound confirmation will be done. An ectopic pregnancy can be identified as early as six weeks from your last menstrual period.

Placental Problems Placental difficulties are a very common indication for sonograms. For example, after twenty weeks of pregnancy, vaginal bleeding may signal the presence of placenta previa. In some cases, women with mild separation of the placenta— which is a potentially serious condition—may also have mild vaginal bleeding, which may be mistaken for placenta previa. Ultrasound helps to make the determining diagnosis.

Diabetics Diabetic mothers usually have several ultrasounds during their pregnancy. The first ultrasound is usually done at twelve weeks. Your physician will want to be assured of three things: the accuracy of your EDD, the baby's normal growth, and the absence of fetal problems. Ultrasounds done later on in pregnancy are used to determine fetal growth, quality of fetal activity, and the amount of amniotic fluid, as well as to check for any abnormalities.

Multiple Pregnancy Knowing early that you will deliver more than one infant gives you time to prepare for the days ahead! An ultrasound ensures that the babies are growing and developing normally and gives you a chance to plan your delivery. Because there is less room inside the womb with a multiple pregnancy, knowing that growth is progressing normally is very important. The ultrasound also indicates the position of the fetuses. One mother talks about her experience:

> I remember that day vividly four years ago when I lay still on the examination table following my ultrasound. I did not move. After having taken the absolute maximum dose of Clomid and Pergonal, I was told that there was a chance that I might have three or more children. My first ultrasound report said that there was a suspicion of more than one baby, but they didn't say how many. This really didn't worry me— I was really more worried that they would have serious medical problems.

Unusual Fetal Positions Ultrasound detects how your baby is situated inside of you. Some caregivers may choose to routinely turn (externally rotate) babies who are in the breech (head up) position, while others believe this is dangerous (see chapter 5). Some say that if the baby is turned during an ultrasound there is minimal risk of problems. The procedure remains controversial and individualized. If the turning is done, it is most often done in a highly controlled situation with an operating room nearby in case immediate delivery is necessary.

Intrauterine Growth Retardation (IUGR) Women at risk for IUGR, such as those with hypertension, kidney disease, heart

disease, placental problems, multiple gestation, infection, poor
weight gain, or the previous birth of a growth-retarded infant,
will usually have more ultrasounds. If you fall into this category,
your physician will do an ultrasound early in your pregnancy and
will follow through with a series of ultrasounds for the duration
of your pregnancy. Usually the ultrasounds are at three-week
intervals. Your baby's head and body measurements and its estimated weight will be taken during each visit. Today, some
women are lucky in being able to know prior to delivery about
the birth of a handicapped child so that they can begin to prepare for the baby's special needs. But often it is difficult to predict the degree of handicap. You should discuss the results of
your ultrasound with your physician and express your concerns
and wishes. A physician may choose to deliver early if the baby
is not growing properly.

Prolonged Pregnancy If you carry your baby past your EDD,
you are considered to have a prolonged or postterm pregnancy.
When your EDD arrives, your amniotic fluid will decrease from
about one quart or 32 oz (1,000 ml) to about 25 oz (800 ml). If
your pregnancy continues, the volume of amniotic fluid may
continue to fall. This decrease is easily detected on the ultrasound. The fetus and placenta also undergo changes associated
with prolonged pregnancy, and in some instances growth may
be halted, a development that may also be identified with
sonography. Ultrasounds are very helpful during the postterm
period because they help identify potential complications
before they arise.

Other Applications Ultrasound may also be done to detect less
common abnormalities such as hydatiform mole. Using ultrasound examination for sex determination is rarely done; however,
if you are having an ultrasound for another reason and you want
to know the sex of your child (which is best seen after twenty-
four weeks), you should feel free to ask. On the other hand, if you
do not want to know, tell the person doing the test at the outset
so that he or she does not blurt it out by accident! You should
know, however, that ultrasound determination of sex is not 100

percent accurate. More women are falsely told they will have a girl than a boy.

What to Expect

Ultrasound may be done either in your physician's office or in the hospital. You may be instructed to drink approximately six glasses of water about one hour before your test. Early in pregnancy, the image of your uterus shows up more clearly on the ultrasound when you have a full bladder. You will probably notice that you will be more uncomfortable during your second ultrasound than your first because of your larger size. Sitting around and waiting for the test will probably be more of a problem than the actual test itself. The discomfort does not last long, and you can urinate as soon as the test is completed.

During your ultrasound you will lie on your back on an examination table. You will be asked to bare your abdomen, and either a gel or an oily substance, serving to improve ultrasound-wave transmission, will be rubbed onto your abdomen. A transducer that is hooked up to a computer screen will be placed on your abdomen, and by looking at the image the transducer produces, the technician or physician will be able to see your baby's status. You can also ask to see your baby and its position.

If an ultrasound is being done before twelve weeks, doctors will often perform a vaginal ultrasound. Using a vaginal transducer, a vaginal ultrasound does not require a full bladder. This procedure is not uncomfortable and provides a better image of the baby.

Special Concerns

Ultrasounds are considered noninvasive, and since their first use in the 1960s no serious hazards have been identified. As in many tests of this type, the results are only as accurate as the person interpreting the data. Ultrasound has opened new horizons in obstetrics, where the well-being of the fetus is always of primary importance. Today, many potential problems are avoided by early detection.

Why Ultrasounds Are Done

Use	Reasons
to estimate fetal age	to time cesareans for those with uncertain dates
to evaluate fetal growth	to ensure good growth
to determine vaginal bleeding	to determine source
to determine fetal position	when difficult to palpate
to determine multiple pregnancy	to monitor pregnancy
during amniocentesis	to ensure correct needle placement
for suspected hydatiform mole	to confirm diagnosis
for suspected cervical incompetence	to measure the cervical length
following cervical cerclage	to aid in timing and correct placement of suture for incompetent cervix
for suspected ectopic pregnancy	to confirm diagnosis
during special procedures	amniocentesis, intrauterine transfusion, IVF, embryo transfer, fetoscopy, CVS
for suspected fetal death	to confirm diagnosis and initiate treatment
for suspected uterine problem	to monitor fetal growth
for ovarian-follicle growth	to determine treatment for infertility
for suspected excessive or insufficient amniotic fluid	to confirm diagnosis and identify cause
if history of previous congenital abnormality	a preventive measure
when turning baby from breech to head-down position	to facilitate safety of procedure
for suspected abruptio placenta	to confirm diagnosis so treatment may be recommended
to screen for abnormalities	routine screening to check growth and development
in prolonged pregnancy	to assess fetal health

EXPANDED AFP SCREENING
(TRIPLE MARKER OR AFP3)

You may be asked if you want to have this optional test. The screening program tests for three different substances using one blood sample: alpha fetoprotein (AFP), human chorionic gonadotropin (hCG), and unconjugated estriol (UE).

The AFP portion of the test checks for neural tube defects. Early in pregnancy this protein is produced by the fetal liver and secreted in the area where the spinal canal, cord, and brain are slowly developing. By the end of the first three months, when the spinal canal is closed, this protein is present in smaller amounts in the amniotic fluid. If present in larger amounts, it may indicate serious disorders such as spina bifida (open spine) or anencephaly (absence of brain). A normal result provides reassurance for the couple that there is little chance of their fetus having either of these problems.

hCG and UE are produced by the woman's placenta and fetus. AFP3 results also provide information regarding the risk of abdominal wall defects, Downs syndrome, and Trisomy 18. Abdominal wall defects occur when a fetus has an abnormal opening on the abdomen allowing the intestines and other organs to form outside of the body. This can be corrected surgically after birth. Downs syndrome is a common cause of mental retardation and heart defects. Low test results may indicate the presence of this defect. An amniocentesis will be done to determine if there is actually a problem. Trisomy 18 is caused by an extra chromosome #18. Babies with this defect suffer from severe mental retardation and usually die before birth or in early infancy.

What to Expect

This test is done by taking a sample of the woman's blood and measuring the amounts of AFP, hCG, and UE. Test results also take into account the mother's age. Because amounts of these substances in the mother's blood change throughout pregnancy, this test is reliable only if performed between fifteen and twenty weeks. Ideally, women should be tested between sixteen and seventeen weeks of pregnancy.

A "screen negative" test result means that the risk for Downs syndrome, Trisomy 18, and neural tube or abdominal wall defects is low and no follow-up tests are necessary. About 90 percent of pregnant women will have a "screen negative" result. A negative result does not mean that the baby will be 100 percent free of birth defects. The AFP Expanded test is a screening program only.

A "screen positive" result reflects an increased risk for one of the birth defects. Follow-up diagnostic tests are offered to determine the reason for a positive test result. If the results indicate a high level of alpha fetoprotein, the test may be repeated in about two weeks. At this time, you should receive genetic counseling and discuss the possibility of an amniocentesis or advanced ultrasound with your genetic counselor or physician. If an ultrasound does not provide an explanation for the initial test result, an amniocentesis will be done.

Special Concerns

The screening program described here is a simple, safe, and relatively reliable group of tests performed by taking a blood sample from the mother's arm. The only disadvantage is that it may provide false positive results. False positive results may be due to a number of reasons, including poor dating of the pregnancy or uncertainty of the date of the last menstrual period. In addition, high levels may be associated with a miscarriage, intrauterine growth retardation, or a multiple pregnancy. Most women who have positive results experience normal follow-up tests and have healthy babies.

According to the Department of Health Services in California, among those who have had the Expanded AFP blood test and follow-up tests in California,

○ 97 percent of the cases of anencephaly are found.

○ 80 percent of the cases of open spina bifida are found.

○ 85 percent of the cases of abdominal wall defects are found.

○ 50 percent or more of the cases of Trisomy 18 are found.

○ 40 percent to 66 percent of the cases of Downs syndrome are found among women age thirty-five and younger.

AMNIOCENTESIS

Amniocentesis is a procedure in which a sample of amniotic fluid is taken from the uterus by inserting a needle through the woman's abdomen into the amniotic sac. It is almost always done using an ultrasound to ensure that the needle is well positioned. The amniotic fluid is then sent to the laboratory for analysis. Amniocentesis is usually done between the fifteenth and eighteenth week of pregnancy, and results usually take between two and three weeks. Early amniocentesis may be performed between the thirteenth and fifteenth week of pregnancy.

Uses

Amniocentesis has many applications. Its most frequent use is for those over the age of thirty-five, to ensure that everything is going well. Other specific applications of amniocentesis include genetic evaluation, checking for metabolic disorders, blood incompatibilities, infection, or neurotube defects, and assessment of fetal lung maturity as the time of birth approaches. If you have been exposed to teratogens (agents that cause birth defects) you may also be advised to have an amniocentesis.

Advanced Maternal Age The purpose of amniocentesis for an older woman is to ensure that there is no sign of genetic abnormalities (see chapters 5 and 14). The procedure is usually done between the fifteenth and eighteenth weeks of pregnancy, early enough for the woman to be able to decide to abort an abnormal fetus.

History of Genetic Problems If there is a history of genetic problems in your family, if you are taking medication for seizures, or if you are an insulin-dependent diabetic, you should be referred for genetic counseling. This counseling will also be recommended if you have had a child with a genetic or chromosomal disorder, such as Downs syndrome, or if either you or your partner carries a recessive trait for a disease.

The cells collected in the amniocentesis sampling can identify the sex of your child. This is important in certain sex-linked

disorders, such as hemophilia, in which females carry the factor
and males manifest the symptoms of the disease.

Metabolic Disorders If your physician suspects a metabolic disorder such as beta-thalassemia or sickle-cell anemia, an amniocentesis may be advised. Beta-thalassemia is a rare metabolic disease, seen most often in Mediterranean regions, that results in
severe anemia in the newborn child. Sickle-cell anemia is seen
most often among the Black population of the United States. In
certain population groups, there may be increased incidence of
Tay-Sachs disease (see chapter 14). This error of metabolism is
characterized by severe neurological problems in the fetus.

During routine prenatal blood testing, high-risk individuals
are screened as carriers of these diseases. If both of the partners
are found to be carriers, an amniocentesis is done to ensure the
baby's health.

Blood Incompatibilities If this is your second pregnancy and you
have had blood incompatibilities with your first child and have
formed antibodies, an amniocentesis may be done to ensure that
your antibodies are not harming your baby-to-be. The amniotic
fluid is analyzed for bilirubin, a yellowish pigment that is formed
as a result of broken-down red blood cells. If the resulting anemia
is harming your unborn child, an intrauterine blood transfusion
may be given so that there may be more safe days for the baby to
mature inside you. When an amniocentesis is done for this reason, it is usually repeated every two to three weeks in order to
detect any possible changes.

Lung Maturity Amniocentesis helps determine the L/S (lecithin/
sphingomyelin) ratio, a ratio that is indicative of fetal lung
maturity—in other words, the fetus's ability to sustain life on its
own. This test is usually done after the thirty-fourth week of gestation and prior to the delivery of a fetus that is not at term but
needs to be delivered as soon as possible. This is also especially
important in the event of premature labor. The test is done to
predict the probability of respiratory distress syndrome (RDS),
which is a common problem among premature babies or babies
born with immature lungs (see chapter 12).

If the test indicates that your baby's lungs are adequately matured, delivery is usually not a problem. However, if the test indicates immature lungs, you may receive an injection of steroid hormone (betamethasone), which helps to facilitate the baby's lung maturation (see chapter 8).

Generally, an L/S ratio of 2.0 indicates that your baby's lungs are mature and that there is a minimal risk of respiratory distress following birth. The results of this particular test will be available the same day of your test, in as little as two to three hours.

A new test is sometimes used instead of L/S ratio, called phoshaltidyl glycerol (PG). It uses the amniotic fluid and takes a little more time to perform.

What to Expect

Amniocentesis for genetic screening is usually done around the fifteen week of pregnancy. It is sometimes also used to check for infection. It may be done either in your physician's office or, more commonly, in genetic centers. You will be told to empty your bladder. Your skin will be cleansed with a special antiseptic solution to prevent infection and then a local anesthetic will be given. During the test, you will lie on your back on the examination table with a sterile cloth placed on your abdomen. The cloth will have a hole in it, through which the needle will pass and enter into your womb. Some women say the injection feels like an insect sting and only lasts a moment.

Guided by the image on the ultrasound screen, the physician will insert the needle into the amniotic sac to obtain a sample of the fluid. The needle insertion sometimes causes uterine contractions. These are usually not serious, and if this does happen your physician will probably wait until the contractions cease before trying again. After the fluid sample is removed, a small bandage is applied. After the test, the fetal heartbeat will be checked to make sure that the procedure was well tolerated. If you are lucky, you may be able to see your baby-to-be move on the ultrasound screen. For most expectant mothers, this is very reassuring and exciting. The actual test takes ten to fifteen minutes; however, you may be asked to remain in the room for about thirty minutes to make sure that both of you are well.

By the time you go home, you should feel normal. If you notice any of the following signs or symptoms, be sure to notify your physician: unusually frequent uterine contractions, abdominal pain, altered fetal activity (more or less), fever, vaginal drainage, or vaginal bleeding. Do not be alarmed by any bruises on your abdomen following the test—they will soon disappear.

Special Concerns

The main concern of an amniocentesis is miscarriage, with a less than 1 percent risk. Only about one in two hundred women experience other side effects, such as cramping, soreness, spotting, vaginal fluid leakage, or infection. Early amniocentesis may pose a higher risk. The decision to have an amniocentesis involves balancing the pros and the cons. The most difficult aspect of having an amniocentesis is having to wait at least two to three weeks for the results.

CHORIONIC VILLI SAMPLING (CVS)

The chorion is the outermost embryonic membrane, which develops about two weeks after fertilization. Eventually it becomes the placenta. An analysis of a sample of this tissue early in pregnancy can detect fetal abnormalities. A decision to terminate the pregnancy may also be made at this point. Although it is no longer used for this reason, CVS was first used in China in 1975 to determine the sex of the child. It has been used in the Soviet Union since 1982 to determine sex-related genetic disorders and continues to be used extensively in other parts of the world.

Uses

The uses of CVS are similar to those of amniocentesis. Certain fetal-blood disorders, such as hemophilia and beta-thalassemia, are also detected in the first trimester by CVS and by fetoscopy. The decision about which procedure to use depends upon the country, the institution, and the physician.

What to Expect

The test is done between the tenth and twelfth weeks of pregnancy. It may be done through the cervix and vagina or the abdomen. Today, the abdominal approach is more common because studies have shown that it has a lower risk of miscarriage. The fetus is first located with an ultrasound. A special needle is inserted through your abdomen, and a small sample of tissue is removed from the placenta. These sample cells, which indicate your baby's genetic composition, are then sent to the laboratory for analysis.

As with an ultrasound, it is important for you to have a full bladder. You may feel a small amount of discomfort as the needle enters the abdomen, and it is normal to spot or bleed slightly after the test. You should report any unusual vaginal leakage or increase in the amount of bleeding.

Special Concerns

While CVS identifies the same defects as amniocentesis, it has some advantages. It can be performed much earlier in pregnancy and the results may be available within one week. Thus, if a major disorder is identified the woman may choose to terminate the pregnancy with a first-trimester abortion.

To date, this procedure is performed only at major medical centers in the United States and may not be available to all women. It is usually recommended to women with problem histories, such as a couple with a Downs syndrome child or another biochemical or genetic problem. The apparent risks of this procedure are slightly greater than those of an amniocentesis. The main risk is miscarriage. Studies have shown that CVS miscarriage rates range from one in two hundred to three in one hundred women (.5 to 3 percent). Women who have had infertility problems may choose not to use this procedure.

PERCUTANEOUS UMBILICAL CORD SAMPLING (PUBS)

This technique, also called funipuncture, involves taking fetal blood samples from the umbilical cord and analyzing the baby's blood cells.

It is performed using ultrasound to guide the needle into the correct location, in the same way as amniocentesis. The fetal umbilical cord is located with the ultrasound, and then a special needle is inserted through the skin into the uterus and into the umbilical cord near the placenta. The ultrasound transducer moves along the woman's abdomen, aiding the physician in finding the umbilical vein. If the fetus is very active a mild sedative may be given so the umbilical cord remains still long enough for the procedure to be done.

This technique may be used later in pregnancy, from about the eighteenth week, to determine the fetus's condition and to identify inherited disorders, such as those detected during amniocentesis. The main advantage of this test is that the results are obtained within one week.

What to Expect

The preparation for this test is similar to that for amniocentesis. Women who are Rh-negative will need an injection of anti-D antibody after this test, in case any fetal cells are disturbed, which could increase the risk of antibody development.

Special Concerns

In many ways, PUBS has gone one step beyond amniocentesis. It tests the fetal blood rather than the amniotic fluid. Today it is considered both diagnostic and therapeutic. For example, if the fetus is ailing due to a blood incompatibility, it may be transfused while in the uterus. In earlier times, these babies would have had to be delivered prematurely.

FETOSCOPY

Fetoscopy is a relatively new procedure, available only in a select number of specialized obstetrical-care centers. The instrument used to perform the test, called a fetoscope, is a telescope or narrow tube about the diameter of a large needle, with a light at the end of it. The fetoscope is inserted through the abdomen in order to view the fetus. The physician is also able to obtain fetal skin or fetal blood samplings through this very fine instrument.

Uses

Some physicians claim that although fetoscopy is a well-established procedure it has limited usage for prenatal diagnosis. It has been used for intrauterine fetal therapy, such as giving blood transfusions, and in identifying defects that are difficult to detect through amniocentesis. The blood samples are used to detect inherited abnormalities, such as sickle-cell anemia, hemophilia, and beta-thalassemia. The results from tests done on samples of blood by fetoscopy are obtained within five days, a quarter of the time it takes for the results of amniocentesis to be processed.

After a possible birth defect is noted via fetoscopy, a physician may choose to do surgery on the fetus using the fetoscope. In some instances, photographs of the fetus may be taken with a special camera located at the end of the fetoscope.

What to Expect

A fetoscopy is often done in the hospital without an overnight stay. Like in amniocentesis, an ultrasound is done before the test to determine fetal age and position. You will have an intravenous drip that may contain a medication to relax you. Prior to the test you will be given a local anesthetic near the site of your incision, which will be very small, about one-eighth of an inch. A tiny tube is inserted alongside the fetoscope to obtain the blood sample. The procedure is usually done between the seventeenth and twentieth weeks, when the blood vessels are mature enough to ensure a sufficient sampling. Fetal skin sampling may also be done on the fetal scalp to detect hereditary skin disorders, although ultrasound directed biopsy has proven to be a safer procedure.

Special Concerns

A fetoscopy is a delicate and costly test that must be done under highly supervised and specialized conditions. It is the only test to date that actually comes into direct contact with the fetus, and this obviously has its risks. With a 5 to 7 percent chance of miscarriage, most consider PUBS to be preferable; however, some claim that this procedure is worth it because of its high accuracy rate.

Salivary Estriol (SalEst)

This test assists physicians in determining risk for spontaneous preterm labor and delivery. The procedure has recently been approved by the FDA for use in women between twenty-two and thirty-six weeks of pregnancy.

The SalEst test measures levels of the hormone estriol in saliva. Studies have shown that the amount of estriol increases dramatically several weeks prior to the onset of preterm labor. This procedure is simple and relatively inexpensive. Patients may collect a small amount of saliva in the physician's office or in their own home. Samples are sent to a lab and results can be obtained within forty-eight hours. The entire process costs around $100. Because the SalEst system is somewhat new, your physician may not prescribe it and certain health plans may not cover the cost. If you would like more information, contact Biex at (800) 404-BIEX.

Fetal Fibronectin (fFN)

The FDA approved the first diagnostic test for predicting a woman's risk for preterm delivery in early 1998. Fetal fibronectin can be used when a woman between twenty-four and thirty-four weeks of pregnancy experiences symptoms of preterm labor. A positive test result acts as a warning signal, alerting the physician that he/she may need to prolong labor using medications, bed rest, or other methods. A negative test result usually means that delivery will not occur within the next seven days. This often allows women to avoid unnecessary treatments. Due to the recent approval of this test, many doctors and insurance companies may not be aware of its existence. Ask your physician or health care provider for more information.

Fetal-Movement Counts

Since biblical times, fetal movements have been viewed as a reassuring sign of a healthy pregnancy. But only in the past few years has the medical community begun to use fetal movements as a serious tool for detecting fetal well-being. This is the only test

	SUN	MON	TUES	WED	THUR	FRI	SAT
9 00		✓					✓
9 30	✓						
10 00			✓		✓		
10 30			✓			✓	
11 00	✓			✓			✓
11 30		✓					
12 00					✓		
12 30						✓	
13 00				✓			
13 30							

Fetal-Movement Graph

that you, the mother, supervise. It is also the test that provides the best indicator of fetal well-being. Most physicians ask at each prenatal visit about the nature of your baby's movements. You should take this question seriously and try to take note of your baby's activity.

Uses

Fetal-movement records are especially important if you are having a difficult or problem pregnancy. Your physician will probably make a special note of the reports you give him or her at each visit. If you say that the movements are less frequent or less intense, further investigations may be done to ensure well-being. A "movement diary" may be recommended from the sixth month onward. Often, babies who are in distress as a result of nutrient or oxygen deficiency in the last trimester of pregnancy tend to slow down or to not move at all.

There are many ways to do a fetal-movement count. Many women find using graph paper to be the simplest method (see the example on page 139). On the top of the page you write the days of the week and on the left you write the time of day. Do the count in the morning or evening, and mark the time you start counting with a check. When you have counted ten movements or kicks, fill in the square corresponding to the time of the last movement. If you do not feel ten kicks in twelve hours, indicate how many you did feel and notify your physician or midwife.

It may be recommended that you count the movements for 60 minutes three times daily, 30 minutes twice daily, 20 to 30 minutes twice daily, 30 minutes a day, or 10 minutes a day. Whatever counting method you are told to use, you should lie on your left side to do the count. It is a good excuse to put your feet up, something pregnant women probably do not get enough time to do!

Special Concerns

The number of kicks felt varies from one woman to another. Some babies seem to be moving all the time, while others are less active. One woman said that with her first pregnancy she had far fewer kicks than with her second. If you do not feel at least ten kicks in two hours, notify your physician or nurse immediately. A nonstress test will probably be recommended.

There are many benefits to the fetal-movement test. One is its low cost and its high reliability—up to 88 percent. It is also simple and safe to do. One disadvantage is that some women tend to panic unnecessarily if they feel that movements are not occurring frequently enough. Remember that babies have patterns of being awake and asleep, just like you do. Studies have indicated that babies are more active at night. Unless you notice a deviation from your baby's normal pattern, it is not necessary to become alarmed. Some may sleep for long periods of time and may have gentle movements. Call your physician or midwife if you have any questions—you owe it to yourself to put your mind at ease!

FETAL MONITORING DEVICES

Today, most women delivering in urban North American hospitals will be exposed to some type of monitoring device. Most hospitals will have you monitored electronically as soon as you are admitted to the maternity unit. There are various types of devices, all with a similar objective of assessing either fetal well-being or uterine contractions. The two most commonly used devices are the fetal stethoscope and the electronic fetal monitor. There are two types of electronic monitors—the internal and the external monitor. Both send information to a machine that records a tracing of the fetus's heart rate and the mother's uterine contractions on graph paper.

The external fetal monitor consists of two small ultrasonic devices strapped around the abdomen; one of them records fetal movements and the other records the muscle tightness of the abdomen or the uterine contractions. The internal fetal monitor consists of an electrode (a small clip) that is inserted vaginally, under sterile conditions, and attached to the scalp of the fetus to measure its heart rate. A tube or catheter is used to measure the strength of the uterine contractions. Although the external fetal monitor is used more often, the internal fetal monitor is more sensitive and can provide important information for a high-risk mother.

The Doppler is another device you may see either on your regular obstetrical visits or during hospitalization. It is used to detect fetal heartbeats using sound waves. The heart rate is counted and recorded by listening to the fetal heartbeat through the abdominal wall. The fetal stethoscope was the only method of assessing fetal heart rate until the advent of portable Doppler machines in the late 1960s.

Although these technological advances help physicians and nurses to keep up with the mother's status minute by minute, it is still common to assess the mother's contractions manually by placing a hand on the fundus (muscular part of the uterus) until a contraction occurs.

Uses

The external fetal monitor is used in both low- and high-risk cases to determine the fetus's status and/or to determine how the baby is handling the stress of labor.

The internal monitoring device is used if external monitoring is not providing the desired results, or if there is a question about fetal well-being. It is only an option if your membranes are ruptured and delivery is expected within a few hours.

The electronic devices are often used for continuous monitoring during hospitalization, either for high-risk situations such as premature rupture of membranes, or during your actual labor. If your condition is stable and the fetal heart rate is stable, your monitor may be removed for a while so that you can get up.

When you are positioned for placement of the electronic monitor, two belts holding two separate devices (a tocotransducer and an ultrasonic transducer) will be placed on your abdomen. They will both be attached to a graph machine that gives a printout of your and your baby-to-be's status. Some women find that these devices restrict their activity because they may need to stay in a certain position to get the best results. Slight movements will show up on the graph, but if they are intermittent they should not affect the results.

Special Concerns

The electronic monitor is accurate in assessing well-being; however, it does restrict your activity, and after each major movement the tocotransducers may have to be readjusted on your abdomen.

TELEMETRY

Telemetry is a new form of continuous fetal monitoring. Unlike the monitoring methods just mentioned, this method allows you to walk about. It basically involves a battery strapped to the thigh that transmits messages from a probe attached to your abdomen or the baby's scalp. It is now readily available in hospitals and works on the same principle as a remote-control television device.

Uses

Telemetry devices have tremendous applications for allowing high-risk women to stay home prior to labor, with continuous monitoring. The woman's status is conveyed via a computer/telephone link to the hospital, usually via an 800-number. Many physicians recommend that the woman at home monitor twice daily, once in the morning and once in the evening.

Telemetry has many advantages, especially that of allowing women to remain at home, reducing the cost of hospital admissions. It is also beneficial for those who travel long distances for their prenatal care.

BIOPHYSICAL PROFILE (BPP)

A biophysical profile (BPP) is a profile that measures the overall fetal well-being, using a scoring system that summarizes the results of other tests that have been done. It is usually done in high-risk pregnancy situations as an additional test. Basically, it relies on an ultrasound and nonstress test to create a profile that provides information such as the amount of amniotic fluid, fetal tone, fetal heart rate, fetal movement, and fetal breathing patterns. Each characteristic is measured on a scale of 0–2, with a total of 10 points indicating the baby is doing perfectly well. If there is a low BPP, the tests will be repeated and the woman will be monitored closely. There is a small risk of false-positive results on this profile.

NONSTRESS TEST (NST)

The fetal nonstress test (NST) assesses your baby's well-being by observing the baby's heart rate in relation to its movements. It is usually not done before twenty-eight weeks except in unusual high-risk situations. It is a noninvasive test done without drugs or anesthesia.

The test involves monitoring the fetal heart rate with a special fetal electronic monitoring device (Doppler). This is on a belt put on your abdomen. The monitor is connected to a machine that looks like a cardiograph machine and makes a printout of the fetal heart rate.

Uses

The nonstress test is usually done in high-risk situations, on women who are being treated for premature labor, multiple pregnancies, decreased fetal movement, postmaturity, or IUGR, or those who are bleeding in their third trimester. Diabetic mothers-to-be as well as those who have preeclampsia and other high-risk conditions will also be candidates for the nonstress test.

What to Expect

This test is fairly straightforward and safe, and it is not painful or uncomfortable. After the monitor is applied, you will be observed for about twenty minutes or until two to five fetal movements or contractions are felt. If none have occurred, you will be observed for another twenty minutes. If they are still not felt, you may be given a snack containing glucose, which often results in an active response. At some point your examiner may choose to stimulate your baby by manipulating your abdomen or ringing a bell to see if there is a response, since fetuses are known to hear sounds from within the uterus. One woman shares this experience:

> After waiting for what seemed like forever, but was only an hour, the nurses decided to excite my baby. I laughed when they walked into my room and dangled a bell over my tummy. I was about six months pregnant, and I think it was the first time I thought of my child as real. It was amazing how quickly my baby responded with kicks. It was within moments of hearing the bell. Of course, I sighed a sigh of relief, as I was sent home because all was well.

Your physician will want to know if your baby is testing reactive or nonreactive. Reactive, which is normal, means that the heart rate speeds up when the baby moves. It is normal for there to be two accelerations, each lasting fifteen seconds or more.

Special Concerns

The most difficult aspect of this test is waiting for fetal movement so that the recording can be completed. The best thing to do if the test lasts longer than anticipated is to be patient and to come with your husband or a friend, or to bring a book or a magazine with you. Another tip to help avoid a lengthy test is to eat prior to the test, since babies are usually more active following meals. Babies born within seven days of a reactive NST are usually in good health.

STRESS TEST

This test, which is seldom done today, has been called the oxy-tocin challenge test (OCT). It has been done in high-risk situa-tions to determine how the fetus reacts during uterine contrac-tions. During careful monitoring, oxytocin, a hormone that stimulates uterine contractions, is given intravenously. The amount of oxytocin injected is increased until there are about three or four contractions in ten minutes (similar to labor). The test takes fifteen to twenty minutes.

Uses

This test helps to determine if the baby can handle the labor process and is used for the same reasons as the nonstress test.

What to Expect

Unlike in the nonstress test, it is a good idea not to eat just prior to the stress test. Nipple stimulation is used first to stimulate labor. This test will be uncomfortable for some, but it is not as uncomfortable as labor. A negative test indicates that the fetus is in good health; a positive test indicates that hospitalization may be necessary. The exact management depends upon how far advanced you are in your pregnancy.

Special Concerns

This test is usually done if a nonstress test provides unclear results. One obstetrician estimated that the ratio of nonstress tests to stress tests being done is about 100:1.

THE ETHICS OF PRENATAL TESTING

The goal of prenatal testing is to detect any problems early, so that they can be diagnosed and treated. For years women went through their entire pregnancy without knowing any details about their baby-to-be. Those who delivered handicapped or deformed babies after nine months of imagining a perfect baby found the shock to be terribly painful. It seems that there is less psychological damage to the mother if she knows early in her pregnancy that she may have a baby with disabilities.

Despite the advantages, the entire area of prenatal diagnosis remains controversial, since there are a number of ethical questions that arise. First, are all these tests necessary, and who decides if they are? The physician? The woman? Or the community as a whole through the establishment of universal criteria? Second, what happens if the tests indicate a problem with the fetus? Who decides what to do? And what happens if there are differing opinions? The issue of abortion emerges.

Difficulties also may occur if you have different beliefs from your physician and/or your spouse. It is important for you to make your wishes known and understood. Remember that it is your body, and your baby-to-be. If you are over thirty-five years of age and your physician does not recommend an amniocentesis, it is your right to ask him or her for one. If you feel that your physician has ordered too many ultrasounds, you should also discuss this with him or her.

Advocates of amniocentesis believe that as a result of prenatal testing there are fewer babies born with serious handicaps than in the past. They argue that the woman now has a choice whether she wants to continue her pregnancy or to abort what tests have shown to be a handicapped child. The opponents of excessive testing argue that the world has gotten along well for countless generations without all this testing and that because many of these tests are new, their long-term effects are yet to be determined.

For some women, it may be difficult to decide whether to have prenatal diagnostic tests. Others undergo testing without thinking twice when they consider that the health of their baby is at stake. The best advice is to be as informed as possible so you can make educated decisions. Be sure that you understand the reasons for the test you are taking and its possible advantages, disadvantages, and risks. Knowledge means confidence, and confidence helps you make the correct decision.

HELPFUL PUBLICATIONS

Good Health Before Pregnancy: Preconceptional Care
Monitoring Fetal Health During Pregnancy
American College of Obstetricians and Gynecologists
Box 4500
Kearneysville, WV 25430-4500

Chapter 8

─────────── ◯ ───────────

Bed Rest and Medications

Most of the treatments for high-risk or problem pregnancies are highly individualized. Chapters 4 and 5 gave an introduction to some of the most common treatments for various types of high-risk pregnancies. This chapter will discuss the role of medications and rest in ensuring a safe pregnancy.

BED REST

Bed rest may be used as a preliminary treatment until the source of your problem is identified. It may also be used as an extended final treatment to prevent premature labor after other treatments have been unsuccessful. The term means different things to different people, and if your physician recommends bed rest you should find out exactly what he or she means. For some it means not getting out of bed at all. For others it may mean having bathroom and dining-room privileges.

Bed rest is often accomplished at home, but in some instances hospitalization may be recommended. Strict bed rest requiring the use of bedpans is prescribed only for a short time following premature rupture of membranes or bleeding from placenta previa. Modified bed rest usually means bed rest with bathroom privileges. If you are required to be on bed rest in the hospital, you will be carefully monitored with either daily or weekly diagnostic tests. Each institution has its own protocol for high-risk mothers. At Parkland Memorial Hospital, a twenty-eight-bed unit in Dallas, for example, women are requested to keep a fetal-movement record by documenting the number of fetal movements for one hour every morning and evening. These records are carefully reviewed by the nurses, and

148

any changes are reported to the physician. Other hospitals will have other protocols.

The following are some common situations in which bed rest may be prescribed.

Threatened Miscarriage

If your pregnancy is threatened you will most likely have some bleeding, and if your physician believes that you are at risk of miscarrying, bed rest may be prescribed. If you have a blighted ovum (see chapter 9), you will miscarry whether or not you are on bed rest. The loss will be due to the malformed egg and not to the level of your activity. If the egg is viable, it is hoped that bed rest will optimize its internal environment and minimize uterine contractions. The length of bed rest depends upon you as an individual, upon your physician, and upon how you feel. Bed rest is sometimes recommended until the bleeding has subsided. Others may recommend it until the end of the first trimester. Remember that your participation in the decision is very important, and you should discuss any of your concerns or questions.

Women with a history of incompetent cervix may be advised to go on bed rest following the surgical placement of cervical cerclage to avoid any strain on the suture. If you are on bed rest for this reason, your physician may prescribe medications to avoid contractions and to decrease the risk of premature labor. These medications are discussed later in this chapter.

Premature Labor

Bed rest is almost always recommended for women going into premature labor, particularly labor prior to the thirty-fourth week of pregnancy. You will probably be advised to lie on your left side, as lying on your back tends to increase uterine contractions and reduce blood flow to the placenta. Those of you who have been pregnant before know about pregnancy-related back problems; lying on your side may help you to avoid them later in your pregnancy. The side-lying position generally improves the blood flow to the uterus while keeping the pressure off the pelvis and cervix. It also may decrease the chances of the cervix dilating and effacing. If you are on bed rest for premature labor, your treatment will probably also include medications to decrease contractions.

Intrauterine Growth Retardation (IUGR)

When your baby's growth lags behind what it should be for its age, your physician might recommend bed rest, specifically lying on your left side, or a reduction in your activity level. A baby that is small for its age is usually associated with a small placenta, and bed rest may increase the blood flow to the placenta, thereby helping the baby to grow properly.

Multiple Pregnancy

Bed rest for the mother facing a multiple pregnancy is a common recommendation, although when it should start and finish is a personal decision made by the caregiver and the woman. The side-lying position is recommended. Some believe that short naps in the morning and afternoon are sufficient, while others might advise modified bed rest to prevent premature labor. Some studies show that bed rest should begin prior to the critical period of twenty-seven weeks and continue until thirty-four weeks. Often bed rest is discontinued when tests show that the fetal lungs are mature enough to sustain life on their own.

Hypertension and Preeclampsia

These diagnoses are often added to other problems associated with high-risk pregnancy, and bed rest may be considered as adjunct therapy to other recommendations. Again, the left side-lying position may help to lower blood pressure problems, because it decreases pressure on the inferior vena cava—the large blood vessel in the back that brings blood back to the heart for oxygenation—and improves blood circulation and urine output.

Pregnant women often feel more tired and find themselves benefiting from a few nap periods a day. The woman who is at high risk for developing elevated blood pressure in pregnancy especially benefits from this extra rest. It is a good idea to have eight to twelve hours of sleep with two nap periods during the day. This may be difficult to manage, especially if you have other children at home, but you should do your best. It may be a good time for your children to learn that there are some things they can do for themselves.

For mild preeclampsia, either bed rest or limited activity is usually advised. In some cases, the physician may choose to admit you to the hospital for close observation. Sometimes women actually request hospitalization, especially if there are other children at home and it is difficult to get rest in the home environment. In most cases, resting is enough to reduce elevated blood pressure.

Heart Disease

Women with a history of cardiac disease may be advised to minimize their activity and/or maintain bed rest, especially in the latter three months of pregnancy, when the strain on the heart is the greatest. If you have heart disease it will be worth investing in well-fitting support hosiery, which help massage the legs and improve blood flow from the legs back to the heart. Many women claim that this hosiery is very comfortable and makes them feel that they have more strength when they are on their feet. In winter months this hosiery provides warmth. Today, support hosiery comes in attractive colors and styles.

Bleeding

Bleeding during either the second or third trimester may be related to a number of factors, including cervical erosion, placenta previa, and abruptio placenta. The placenta is most often the source of such bleeding. Bed rest may be recommended to minimize the bleeding, and sometimes a stay in the hospital is advised until the bleeding subsides. The effects of bed rest are augmented by a relaxing and calming environment. Studies have shown that increased activity and even sensory stimulation may actually increase bleeding. Sometimes the best place to rest is in the hospital.

Premature Rupture of Membranes

This is a condition that demands careful attention. If your membranes rupture prematurely, the first recommendation you will receive is to maintain complete bed rest to prevent excessive drainage of amniotic fluid. After about twelve to twenty-four hours your physician may allow you to walk to the bathroom rather than using a bedpan. Often a woman who has premature rupture of the membranes is hospitalized; however, if you are sent home, you may be instructed to stay quiet and not to plan too much activity. You should clarify this recommendation with your physician, but do yourself and your baby a favor—take it easy!

It is important to avoid any chance of infection after the membranes have ruptured. Intercourse is not recommended. You should take only showers, and monitor your temperature in the morning and evening. If you find that it is over 100°F (38°C), notify your physician as soon as possible. With these safety measures, chances are that you will successfully carry your baby without problems.

COPING WITH BED REST

Bed rest is not fun at the best of times, nor is it an absolute cure for any high-risk problem. The emotional adjustment to bed rest may be very difficult, especially if you lead an active life, working full-time at home or at a career. Becoming dependent when you are used to being independent is never easy, and you may find that the smaller things in life, like phone calls and the mail delivery, will become the highlights of your day!

If you have other children at home, it may be difficult for them to understand your inactivity. When I was on bed rest with my second pregnancy, my two-year-old, who enjoyed being held, could not understand why I was no longer able to lift her. She was deeply hurt, feeling that I did not love her anymore, and had great difficulty coping. She used various types of attention-seeking behaviors to test my love for her. I made a point of sitting on the floor with her and hugging her at her level. This meant a lot to her—as most parents will agree, there can never be enough hugging.

Another woman with an older child comments:

Joan was seven years old when I was told I would have to be on bed rest with my second child. Somehow it wasn't much of a problem, because she was already established in school and the school bus picked her up and dropped her off each day. As a matter of fact, I think she liked having me on bed rest because it was probably the only time, both before and after the pregnancy, that she knew where to find me. I was simply always in bed and there when she needed me.

Your partner will also feel burdened with more responsibilities and may feel intense pressure at times. Many women sense feelings of resentment from their spouses. It is normal for him to lose patience with you, because he will be under an enormous amount of pressure. Try to be patient and loving during these times and keep communication channels open.

My husband was very strong during my pregnancies, offering ongoing love and respect. Understandably, there were days when the tension got to him, especially toward the latter part of the pregnancy. I often wondered if I would have been as intensely patient and loving as he was.

Adequate support systems are important during this time. If you are able, you should seek home-care help to assist you and your family. People who will clean and do the shopping are invaluable. A list of students who can run errands may be helpful if you live in a school community. Remember that even though you are on bed rest, you can continue to manage your household.

Keeping busy is often difficult for the bedridden mother-to-be. Try to contact other mothers who have been on bed rest and ask how they spent their time. This will not only offer you tips but will also boost your confidence. Inquire about home manicures, massages, hairstyling, and other pampering and relaxing activities. This is also a good time to catch up on reading, knitting, sewing, writing, and other hobbies that you used to say you never had time for. Listening to calm music is also good for both you and your baby.

Mental rest is as important as physical rest for the high-risk mother. You should have a relaxing environment with quiet diversional activities. Any concerns you have should be voiced.

Most important, remember that you are in bed not because you are sick but because you are awaiting the birth of your child.

Passive Exercises for Bed Rest

Kegel Exercises Lie on your back or sit up. Tighten your pelvic floor muscles (as if stopping your urine). Hold for three counts, then relax.

Abdominal Breathing Lie on your back with knees bent and breathe in deeply, letting your abdominal wall rise. Exhale slowly through your mouth as you tighten your stomach muscles.

Bridging Lie on your back with your knees bent. Raise your hips off the bed while keeping your shoulders down.

Curl-ups Lie on your back with knees bent. Put your hands on your stomach. Lift your head and shoulders up (touch your chin to your chest), keeping the small of your back against the bed.

Leg Sliding Lie on your back with your knees bent. Slide your legs out, slowly straightening your knees against the bed. Slowly pull both knees back up.

Modified Leg Raises Lie on your back with one knee bent. Bend the other knee up toward your chest, then straighten your leg by kicking up toward ceiling, and then lower your leg to the bed. Repeat with the other leg.

Abduction Lie on your back with knees bent. Let your knees come apart, then squeeze them back together.

Ankle Circles Lift your ankles up and down. Rest your right ankle on your left knee and circle in both directions. Repeat with the left ankle on the right knee.

Arm Lifts Exhale deeply through your nose as you lift one arm up to the side over your head. The sides of your chest should expand. Exhale as you bring your arm down. Repeat with the opposite arm.

MEDICATIONS

Any medications used during pregnancy should be taken with extreme caution. The best attitude while pregnant is that drugs and other medications should not be taken unless prescribed. Do not take any over-the-counter medications without consulting your physician: what may ordinarily be a harmless medication could be a potential hazard for you and/or your baby. For example, aspirin is not recommended for extensive use because it interferes with blood clotting. Your baby is most vulnerable during the first three months when the body's structures are formed and defects are likely to occur. Remember that while you are caring for yourself you must also care for the needs and requirements of your baby.

Medications That May Be Hazardous to the Fetus

Category	Example
analgesics	aspirin, advil
antibiotics	tetracycline, doxycline
anti-blood-clotting medications	warfarin
antidepressants	lithium, imipramine, MAO inhibitors
antiseizure medications	phenytoin
cancer-fighting medications	methotrexate
hormones	diethylstilbestrol (DES), synthetic progesterone, testosterone
tranquilizers	diazepam

There are some medications that the high-risk mother may take for the treatment of certain pregnancy-related problems. Although there may be side effects associated with some of them, they are usually prescribed because the benefits for the baby far outweigh the risks. Have faith in your physician: it makes a difficult pregnancy much easier. If you do not have faith, get more information or change physicians.

Some Medications Used in High-Risk Pregnancy

Drug	Use
Albuterol	labor suppressant
Aldomet	hypertension
Apresoline	hypertension
Betamethasone	fetal-lung maturity
Ergotrate sulfate	uterine stimulant
Indomethacin	labor suppressant
Magnesium sulfate	labor suppressant, preeclampsia
Nifidipine	labor suppressant
Pitocin	uterine stimulant
Prostaglandins	uterine stimulant
Prostaglandin inhibitors	labor suppressant
Rh immune globulin	Rh incompatibility prevention
Ritodrine hydrochloride	labor suppressant
Syntocinon	labor stimulation

Labor Suppressants

These medications are prescribed for premature labor prior to the thirty-sixth week. Taking them will give your baby an increased chance to grow and mature inside you. Labor suppressants are rarely given if your membranes have ruptured prematurely; if they are, it is usually in conjunction with steroid therapy. Some common types of labor suppressants include beta-adrenergic receptor stimulants, such as ritodrine (Yutopar), terbutaline sulfate (Brethine), indocin (Indomethacin), and magnesium sulfate.

Beta-Adrenergic Medications Ritodrine was first approved by the FDA in 1980. It is probably the newest labor suppressant and is administered after the twentieth week and prior to the thirty-fifth week to prevent preterm labor. Some women, such as those with an incompetent cervix, take ritodrine or Vasodilan orally starting in early pregnancy to prevent uterine contractions. If active preterm labor has begun, the drug may be given intravenously in the hospital, and if labor is stopped you may be sent home on bed rest with the oral form. Today, women are given home monitors to check contractions several times each day.

Recent innovations, including the development of the continuous infusion pump, help provide a constant low level of the medication in the bloodstream. The use of this device is usually prescribed with terbutaline when oral medications do not control labor and prolonged hospitalization is not favorable.

Beta-adrenergic medications are usually continued until the thirty-seventh week. They are generally considered quite safe for the developing fetus, though some claim that they may increase the baby's heart rate or lower its blood sugar levels. Babies are usually carefully assessed for these side effects following delivery.

Mothers may experience any of the following side effects: mild tremors, nausea, headaches, hypertension, drowsiness, urinary incontinence, lowered blood pressure, or elevated blood sugar levels. Although dosage adjustment is rarely necessary, you should inform your physician about any of these effects. Sometimes routine potassium checking may be necessary, or the addition of potassium-rich foods such as bananas and dried fruits may be recommended.

Ritodrine is the medication that I took with my second and third pregnancies. I found the side effects to be minimal, at least less bothersome than those associated with Vasodilan, which I took during my first pregnancy. On occasion you may feel your heart beating rapidly. Although I never experienced other symptoms, some women complain of nausea, sweating, and headaches.

Terbutaline sulfate, which is very similar to ritodrine, has been successful in suppressing labor by relaxing the uterine muscles and decreasing the pressure inside the uterus. Some women have reported side effects such as nervousness, headaches, increased maternal and fetal heart rate, and muscle cramps. These may be related to the dosage and may not occur on small or moderate doses of this medication. Terbutaline is administered with a portable external infusion pump, which was originally designed for insulin administration. This medication can be started as an IV or subcutaneous dose in the hospital. You may then be sent home with oral medication.

Magnesium Sulfate This medication was first used nearly fifty years ago for severe preeclampsia to prevent seizures, and only recently has it been used to treat preterm labor. It is given only in the hospital, by injection. As with most medications, there are side effects, including nervousness, breathing difficulties, flush-ing, warmth, altered heart rate, and changes in muscle reflexes. The most serious side effect is pulmonary edema (water in the lungs), seen in about 2 percent of women. However, some believe that this medication has fewer side effects than others, and it is therefore the medication of choice in high-risk pregnancy. In addition, it is relatively safe for the baby—side effects are rare. Following delivery, babies are monitored for lower calcium levels and decreased muscle tone.

Nifidipine/Procardia This is a relatively new medication, first used to treat those with an irregular heartbeat and now used to decrease uterine contractions. It works by interfering with the action of calcium, which plays a major role in muscle contrac-tions. Women who cannot tolerate terbutaline are often pre-scribed nifidipine. It may also be used in conjunction with terbu-taline. Side effects can include dizziness, headache, and lowered blood pressure. Some doctors recommend that patients chew the capsule to break it up before swallowing.

Indomethacin This medication is a prostaglandin inhibitor and is used prior to the thirty-fourth week. It has been found to be very effective in stopping preterm labor, with only rare side effects to the mother. Long-term use of this drug may result in a decrease in amniotic fluid and/or possible heart, lung, digestive, or kidney problems for the baby. Usually this medication should not be taken more than forty-eight hours at a time. For these reasons, most health-care providers consider Indomethacin a second-line medication.

Special Concerns Because most of these medications cause an ele-vated heart rate, depending upon the dosage prescribed, it is a good idea to take your pulse at the same time each day to ensure that your dosage is properly adjusted. Most health-care providers expect your pulse to be between 95 and 105 per minute, but you should notify your caregiver if it rises over 125. You should report any complaints of chest pain or shortness of breath. Also, you should notify your provider of any feelings of nervousness, agitation, and/or tremors. This may mean your dosage needs to be adjusted.

Uterine Stimulants

Uterine stimulants are used to initiate or augment the labor process. They are used for a variety of reasons, such as to induce labor, to offset the effects of postmaturity on your baby, for blood incompatibilities and fetal-growth impairment, and to strengthen uterine contractions in long labors. Some practitioners prescribe medications alone to induce labor, while others prefer to manually rupture the membranes. For labor induction to be successful, a woman must be toward the end of her pregnancy and her cervix must be thin, soft, and somewhat dilated. The most common type of uterine stimulant is oxytocin (prepared synthetically as pitocin and syntocinon). Prostaglandins or misoprostil are sometimes used to prepare the cervix and induce labor.

Pitocin and Syntocinon Oxytocin is a natural hormone, secreted by the pituitary gland, that stimulates uterine muscle contractions. It is injected into the bloodstream in very low doses and under highly supervised hospital conditions at the time of labor and delivery. Some women note side effects such as anxiety, lower blood pressure, increased heart rate, and excessive uterine contractions. Because it is administered in the hospital, where the side effects may be detected and reported early, there are rarely any long-term risks.

Prostaglandins These are naturally occurring hormone-like substances present in various parts of the body. When used to induce labor, they block the release of two hormones—progesterone and relaxin—from the ovaries and stimulate uterine contractions. Prostaglandins are most often used to induce abortion in early stages of pregnancy, since their side effects, such as nausea, vomiting, and diarrhea, may be extreme later in pregnancy. They are sometimes also given prior to induction to soften or mature the cervix. A relatively new type of induction procedure uses prostaglandin gel, applied directly to the cervix to help soften it and to stimulate the labor process. A new medication, called Misoprostil, is used in a similar manner.

What to Expect During Induction   Prior to being induced, you will be connected to the fetal monitor (see chapter 7) and the uterine-contraction monitor for careful surveillance. You will be on your left side and will have an intravenous drip containing the pitocin/syntocinon solution. The goal of the induction is for you to have uterine contractions every two to three minutes lasting forty-five to sixty seconds. Labor may be induced over two days, allowing you to rest overnight between inductions. The induction will be stopped immediately if there is any sign of you or your baby being in danger.

Special Concerns   Women are induced for a variety of reasons. Sometimes inducing labor is done for "social" reasons—for the convenience of either the woman or the physician. This is condemned by many people. Five or ten years ago, women who had previous cesareans would not be induced. Today, these women are treated more and more like those with normal pregnancies, and they might be induced if needed. Women who are induced because of postmaturity are often relieved that their pregnancy is coming to an end. For some, the induction process may be frightening. Some women fear having stronger and more painful contractions with artificially induced labor. Actually, stimulated labor is similar to normal labor, accompanied by even more careful monitoring.

One mother comments on her induction:

> I was induced with my first child at forty-two weeks primarily because I had a slow leak of amniotic fluid and vague contractions. There was some confusion as to the baby's position. What they thought was the head was actually her shoulder. She was in the transverse position. I was put on a syntocinon drip for twelve hours with no results. Labor was not progressing. I remember becoming nervous at one point because the fetal heart rate doubled and there was meconium. The baby was in distress, and they finally did an emergency cesarean. These scary moments passed when I was suddenly consoled by the birth of a beautiful healthy baby girl.

Babies are being born today that would not have survived years ago. It is true that some of the medications discussed have side effects, but the benefits in most situations far outweigh the risks.

Chapter 9

―――――――――――――― ◯ ――――――――――――――

Miscarriage

A miscarriage, sometimes called a spontaneous abortion, is the spontaneous termination of a pregnancy prior to the twentieth week of gestation. An "early" miscarriage occurs prior to twelve weeks of gestation, and a late miscarriage occurs between the twelfth and twentieth weeks. Nearly 15 percent of all pregnancies result in miscarriage, most often during the first three months of pregnancy, making it the most common type of pregnancy loss. Many miscarriages are not even recognized because they happen so early.

Miscarriages are not discussed very often, since they are considered a "normal" variation of the gestational process. Many women also prefer not to talk about a miscarriage because of its personal nature and the accompanying feelings of failure and loss. For them, this can be a lonely time. Other women say that they never realized how many women have miscarriages until they start speaking to others about it. As one woman says,

> After I miscarried, it seemed as if everyone I spoke to either had had a miscarriage or knew someone who did. It was unbelievable. It certainly helped me feel less alone knowing that other women knew what I was going through. It didn't take the pain away, but it certainly facilitated the grieving process.

Without question, miscarriage has a strong emotional and physical impact on a woman. How she copes with this tragedy will depend on how she has coped with other traumas in her life. Even for the strongest person, the loss of a baby is psychologically and emotionally very difficult. Both partners feel the impact deeply. People who have never experienced a miscarriage often do not see it as the death of a baby, and may regard it as a rather common occurrence. Thus the grief a couple feels is often downplayed by those who do not understand what they are going through.

There are many reasons for miscarriage, which have been discussed in detail earlier. The exact cause is usually difficult to establish unless you have a structural abnormality in the reproductive system that is well documented through tests such as the hysterosalpingogram, or have had an infection that was not adequately treated.

WHAT HAPPENS

Not all women have warnings before their miscarriage. The earliest sign is vaginal bleeding, ranging from a heavy flow to a few drops every few hours, during the first three months of pregnancy. The spotting is initially dark, as progesterone and estrogen levels decrease, causing the endometrium to slough. It may then turn to pink or bright red, as the blood vessels open and the products of conception begin to separate. One woman remarks,

> It was the most unusual thing. We were sitting down to have a quiet supper one evening, when I was exactly three months pregnant. Suddenly I got abdominal cramping as if I had some form of food poisoning. I immediately went to the bathroom and was lucky I did, because right there I began losing what seemed like an enormous amount of blood. I sat on the toilet and could feel the fetal products leaving me, forever. We went right to the hospital and I had a D&C. It all happened so quickly.

Another woman recalls the following experience:

> I denied everything that was happening to me. I spotted on and off during the first three months. I vividly remember one day at work when I spotted more than usual. I called my obstetrician and he advised me to go home immediately. He suggested that it may or may not be serious but advised bed rest until the bleeding stopped. It took about three days for the bleeding to stop, and since the third day landed on a

Friday, I decided to also spend the weekend in bed—just to ensure that all was well.

Everything was fine for the weekend and I returned to work on Monday. I saw my obstetrician on Tuesday for a checkup and all was well. Thursday night I was having intense abdominal cramps accompanied by heavy bleeding and went immediately to the emergency room. I lost my baby in the hospital. It was the most traumatic experience in my life.

Cramping and vaginal bleeding during pregnancy sometimes indicates that a miscarriage is occurring. You should save all tissue and products that you pass and bring them either to your physician's office, if it is during office hours, or to your local hospital's emergency room. You may want to phone first to ask where you should go in order to avoid any unnecessary running around. When the physician sees you, you will probably have an examination with a speculum to try to determine the source of your bleeding. You may also have tests such as ultrasounds to assess your baby's status. If you do miscarry, your breasts may also begin to feel less tender and less full. After the miscarriage has occurred, some physicians recommend doing certain blood tests or even an endometrial biopsy. The blood sample will be analyzed for various hormonal levels, which may give your physician a clue as to the cause of your miscarriage.

TYPES OF MISCARRIAGES

There are several types of miscarriages, some of which require more medical attention than others.

Threatened Miscarriage

This refers to any bleeding or spotting in early pregnancy, which may or may not be associated with cramping or back discomfort, indicating that a miscarriage may occur. The continuation of your pregnancy is usually in doubt. It may be an uneasy time, because you do not know whether to plan for your baby or not. Everything seems to be up in the air. Your physician will probably recommend

restricted activity, bed rest, no douching or tampons, and abstinence from intercourse for anywhere from a few days to two
weeks after bleeding begins. If your cervix is open, your chances
of infection will be increased. Also, having anything inside the
vagina may trigger uterine contractions.

Inevitable Miscarriage

This refers to a pregnancy termination that is actually in progress
and cannot be stopped. Symptoms include bleeding and pain that
may be cramplike in the beginning and then become more
intense. The cervix dilates or the membranes of the amniotic sac
break, resulting in a gush of amniotic fluid expelled from the
vagina, and then there are contractions and expulsion of fetal
components. Your physician will probably recommend bed rest
for forty-eight hours. If bleeding continues and/or fever develops,
a D&C will most likely be done.

Incomplete Miscarriage

This is when the fetus and placenta are not completely expelled
from the uterus and bleeding may be very heavy. A D&C is necessary to remove the placental tissue. Incomplete miscarriages
generally occur after twelve weeks of pregnancy.

Missed Miscarriage

A missed miscarriage is an unpleasant circumstance in which the
first twelve weeks progress normally, and then the fetus dies and
remains in the uterus for four or more weeks without the woman
feeling any pain or bleeding. Some women complain of intermittent vaginal bleeding or brownish discharge.

Symptoms include an obvious decline in uterine growth and
lack of fetal development. Your breasts also return to their normal size. Eventually, the fetus aborts. If it does not, you may
develop serious blood abnormalities and a D&C may be necessary. It is best to have a D&C as soon as it is established that the
fetus has died. The longer you wait, the greater are your chances
of getting a uterine infection or a condition called disseminated

intravascular coagulation (DIC), a serious problem. It is also better for you to terminate your relationship with your fetus, because
psychologically it can be very draining to carry a dead fetus.

Habitual Aborter

A habitual aborter is a woman who has a series of miscarriages.
This may indicate a hidden problem of either fetal, genetic, or
maternal origin. Some medical authorities say that two or more
miscarriages are considered habitual, while others believe that
three or more put a woman in this category. Once the problem is
diagnosed and treated, however, 70 to 80 percent of women can
be cured. Some possible causes of habitual abortion include
incompetent cervix, chromosomal disorder, immunological problems, uterine defect, and hormonal imbalance.

If you have had many miscarriages after sixteen weeks of
pregnancy, your physician will probably suspect an incompetent
cervix. If a chromosomal disorder is suspected, you and your partner may need to be evaluated genetically. If hormonal imbalance
is your problem, your physician may recommend hormonal suppositories, such as progesterone, which are usually started at the
time of ovulation and continue until the twelfth to fourteenth
week of gestation (others may begin it as soon as you have a positive pregnancy test). Some may choose to give progesterone or
hCG injections at the first sign of bleeding and once more two
weeks later.

THE EMOTIONAL IMPACT OF MISCARRIAGE

Miscarriage is an event that affects both members of the couple—
though the actual impact is almost always different for each
member, which often results in additional stress. This is because
the bonding that occurs is different for men than it is for women.

Although having a miscarriage is very scary, it is rarely life-
threatening today, and the most difficult part is the aftermath.
When a woman's body heals and she goes home without her
baby, she is often overwhelmed by grief and sadness. It may
seem to her like everything is coming to an end. In addition to
the emotional impact of losing a baby, her hormones are also

returning to their pre-pregnant state and depression may accompany this adjustment.

After a miscarriage you may experience emotions such as anger and disappointment at having lost the baby, and guilt about whether you caused it. These feelings are all normal and are part of accepting your loss. You may become angry with yourself and with those around you. This anger is marked by questions such as "Why me?" If you have had more than one miscarriage, you may begin to wonder why pregnancy is so easy for some and so difficult for you. One obstetrician says that although most of his patients have "accepted it as a fact of life," many feel "it was my fault. I should have taken better care of myself." Sometimes the guilt is magnified by other people's comments. One woman remarks:

> I'll never forget my sister's comments when she phoned me at home following the miscarriage. Her exact words were "Maybe they made a mistake; maybe it really wasn't a miscarriage." I couldn't believe what she was telling me. She was denying that anything happened to me and here I was absolutely devastated. Nobody would let me grieve. Nobody seemed to understand that I was experiencing an enormous amount of emotional pain.

Another woman shares her experience:

> I remember trying to open up to an orderly who was looking after me in the hospital. I always related better to men. I broke down in tears when we spoke. The next thing I knew, he was asking me if I was religious because I was so upset. I was so insulted.

Guilt feelings may be very strong in some women and may last for many years after the miscarriage. If you have any guilt feelings, it is best to verbalize them with your loved ones rather than keeping them pent up inside you. Another alternative would be to seek professional one-on-one counseling to discuss what you are going through.

Some couples find it very easy to speak about their loss, while others find it very difficult. Support groups can be encouraging for those who feel comfortable in group situations. If you want to share what you have been through and are more comfortable in a one-on-one situation, ask about the services offered in your hospital, such as those provided by social workers.

Everyone reacts differently to the loss. Some women say that each time they see an infant, they burst into tears. You may find yourself avoiding visits or contact with women who have babies. You may find that you break down each time you hear a baby cry. You may be filled with unrelenting pent-up emotions—emotions that you never thought existed inside of you. One woman comments,

> Others who have never had a miscarriage really don't understand what a woman goes through. I remember people questioning my grief the following week. My own sister couldn't understand why I was still so emotionally upset. Most people expect women to just shake the event—however, in reality, this is impossible.

Socializing following a miscarriage may be difficult, especially during the immediate mourning period. It may be best to integrate yourself gradually with those around you, starting with those who are closest to you and then expanding to less familiar people.

It is normal for your grief to take you by surprise. You may think you have rid yourself of the grief, only to find yourself breaking down crying unexpectedly some time after the loss. This hypersensitivity varies from one person to another and may last days, weeks, months, or years. This mourning period is considered healthy, and it helps to heal the wounds of the loss. As one woman who had three miscarriages states,

> It's amazing how we hear only what we want to hear. I remember blocking out all the negative situations or problems during my childbirth-education classes. They told us all about miscarriage, stillbirth, and even neonatal death. It is as if I don't remember a thing about what they said. After I miscarried, I tried to mobilize the information I learned at these classes and my mind went completely blank.

Essentially, the loss you and your partner feel is the loss of a child you never knew. It is particularly difficult if you have been trying for a long time to become pregnant. In their book *Coping with Miscarriage*, Christine Palinski and Hank Pfizer say that the fear takes two forms—agony over the chances for subsequent pregnancies to succeed, and the fear that the physician would say that something even more terrible (perhaps life-threatening) than miscarriage was occurring.

Deciding when to become pregnant again is often a difficult and frightening choice for the couple. Some say that the right time to become pregnant is when you feel ready—that is, when you and your partner have acknowledged that the miscarriage was not your fault and was beyond your control. This often means that the mourning period is essentially completed.

While 70 to 90 percent of women who miscarry eventually become pregnant again, there is a 15 to 20 percent chance of having a subsequent miscarriage. If your previous pregnancy was the result of months of temperature charts and infertility work-ups, the thought of reliving that laborious process may not be very tempting.

You waited so long for that pregnancy—and now you are back to square one. You may become impatient with yourself and with your partner, but it is very important for both of you to be sensitive to each other, tolerant, and accepting. You should wait three months before trying to get pregnant again. The key is not to worry about the chance of having a miscarriage. As one obstetrician put it, "You cannot live your life in fear."

Coping with Miscarriage

○ Speak with other women who have miscarried.

○ Join miscarriage support groups or private counseling.

○ Communicate openly and honestly with your partner.

○ Be patient with yourself.

○ Spend time with those close to you.

○ Cry if you feel like crying.

○ Remember that 15 percent of all pregnancies end in miscarriage; you are not alone.

○ Wait at least three months before becoming pregnant again.

HELPFUL PUBLICATIONS

Empty Arms: Coping After Miscarriage, Stillbirth and Infant Death
    by Sherokee Ilse
Order from:
Wintergreen Press
3630 Eileen Street
Maple Plain, MN 55359
(612) 476-1303

Chapter 10

———————— ◯ ————————

Other Losses

The loss of a baby may be less common today then it was five or six decades ago, but it is no less painful. If you have had a high-risk pregnancy, you probably thought about the possibility of the death of your child. These fears are perfectly normal. It is healthiest in the long run to discuss them with your husband, a friend, a relative, or your childbirth educator. Some women may detach themselves from the loss of their child, and this may result in unresolved grief. These denied feelings will unexpectedly surface later.

No matter how prepared you are, when your baby dies you will experience a wide range of emotions, including shock, despair, and frustration. This is especially true if getting pregnant was difficult and/or if this pregnancy and previous ones were complicated. You will want to hold on to that baby's life and you may find yourself denying the loss.

A baby may die at any point during pregnancy or immediately afterward. Researchers believe that the effects of loss are in direct proportion to the closeness of the relationship prior to death. The five most common types of loss during pregnancy and immediately afterward include abortion, miscarriage, stillbirth, neonatal death, and sudden infant death syndrome.

ABORTION

Abortion is an option for unwanted pregnancies, and in the event of certain fetal problems. Today, prenatal diagnosis is primarily performed so that in the event of a fetal problem, the woman has the option to terminate her pregnancy. Some possible situations include those women who have a medical problem, those who contracted rubella (German measles) early in pregnancy, those exposed to environmental hazards such as radiation, toxic chemicals, or certain medications, and those carrying a baby with a genetic disorder.

The Decision

Most of the tests that indicate that a fetus has abnormalities are done in the fourth month, and in many cases this is after a woman has begun to feel her baby move. It is very difficult to make the decision to terminate a pregnancy once this sign of life has been felt. Deciding the fate of a fetus can be an awesome responsibility. Couples choose prenatal tests for a variety of reasons. Some choose them for reassurance (about 98 percent of the results are normal), others if they suspect fetal problems. Some couples choose not to have the procedures because they have no intention of having an abortion, while other couples are very sure that they would be unable to devote their lives to raising a child with disabilities. Others use the knowledge gained from these tests to help them prepare for a child who may require specialized care. Those less sure probably find the decision-making process most difficult of all.

Some hospitals have counselors who are specially trained to assist people in coming to terms with their decision. If you and your partner do not know what to do and want to know the options, you may benefit from speaking to these professionals. They will not make your decision for you, but they may offer you another perspective that will help you come to terms with your situation.

What to Expect

The method of abortion used depends upon your stage of pregnancy. There are three abortion procedures: dilation and curettage (D&C), dilation and evacuation (D&E), and induction.

Dilation and curettage involves dilating the cervix and scraping the contents of the uterus. This is usually done in the first twelve weeks of pregnancy and is done under local or general anesthesia.

Dilation and evacuation involves dilation, suction, curettage, and the use of forceps to evacuate the uterine contents. This is usually done between twelve and twenty-four weeks of pregnancy, and it may also be done under either local or general anesthesia. Many claim that the D&E has advantages over the induction methods (see below) used in the second trimester. The D&E is safer and physically and emotionally easier for a woman. It is also quicker (ten to forty minutes) compared to the overnight stay required with an induction abortion. A D&E may be done in the physician's office or in a clinic. Many physicians may feel uncomfortable removing a fetus at this stage of development, however, and may opt for induction abortions.

An induction abortion, sometimes called an instillation procedure, saline abortion, or prostaglandin abortion, is done only after the sixteenth week of pregnancy, because the amniotic sac is not large enough to be located accurately until this time. The procedure is done by injecting certain chemicals, such as a saline solution or the hormone prostaglandin, through the abdomen into the amniotic sac to induce labor. Hours later, uterine contractions will cause the cervix to dilate and the fetus and placenta will be expelled. The induction of labor may take anywhere from twenty-four hours to a few days, and this waiting period may be very difficult. Some centers choose to do a vaginal application of prostaglandin at fourteen to twenty weeks instead of using the abdominal method. A vaginal suppository is given that stimulates uterine contractions and the expulsion of the fetus and placenta. A D&C is sometimes also done.

Before having your D&C, you will have a bimanual exam to feel the size of your uterus and determine your stage of pregnancy. Then a speculum will be inserted into your vagina. You may feel some pressure, but this should not hurt. Your vagina will be cleaned to prevent infection and, if you consent, a local anesthetic will be injected into the cervix. Since the cervix has only a few nerve endings, you may only feel a pinch. An instrument will be inserted to keep the cervix steady, and the cervical opening will be gradually stretched. You may feel some mild cramping, similar to menstrual cramps. A strawlike tube or cannula is inserted through the cervix and connected to a bottle, which is connected to a vacuum pump. A gentle suction will remove the pregnancy tissue. The aspiration takes only a few minutes, depending upon how pregnant you are. You may feel some cramping, which should subside shortly after the cannula is removed.

Before you leave, you may feel weak, tired, and nauseated for a while. Your counselor will give you instructions on what to watch for, such as increased bleeding or cramping.

Having an abortion does not decrease the chance of having a healthy baby in the future. Some studies have indicated that repeated abortions may slightly increase the chances of miscarriage and premature birth because repeated dilations of the cervix may, in some women, weaken the muscle.

Your Emotions

Positive, negative, and mixed emotions are all very common following an abortion. For some, the abortion may provide relief of an unwanted pregnancy. You and your partner will probably feel that it is the right decision for you at this time. Knowing that it is the right decision, however, does not give immunity from the emotional impact of the experience. Feelings of guilt are common and may be reinforced by the discomfort you feel after the actual procedure. You may wonder once again if it was the right decision, what the child may have looked like, and the effect it could have had on your life. These questions must remain unanswered, but the most difficult and the most important question has been answered and you should have the confidence to agree that it was the right decision.

Recovering from an abortion is not easy. As Rayna Rapp said in a *Ms.* article entitled "The Ethics of Choice,"

> Recovering from the abortion took a long time. Friends, family, coworkers, and students did everything they could to ease me through the experience. Even so, I yearned to talk with someone who'd "been there." Over the next few months, I used my personal and medical networks to locate and talk with a handful of other women who'd opted for selective abortions. In each case, I was the first person they ever met with a similar experience. The isolation of this decision and its consequences is intense. Only when women (and concerned men) speak of the experience of selective abortion as

tragic but chosen fetal death can we as a community offer support, sort out the ethics, and give the compassionate attention that such a loss entails.

STILLBIRTH

A stillbirth is the birth of a fetus that has died at any time after twenty weeks of pregnancy. There are several possible causes of stillbirth. Rare, unexplained blood clots may form in the umbilical cord, preventing oxygen from getting to the baby, or the placenta may prematurely separate from the baby, cutting off its oxygen. About 5 to 10 percent of all stillbirths are due to chromosomal abnormalities or congenital deformities. If you have a history of stillbirths and early miscarriages, your physician may recommend genetic screening to rule out any genetic problem in either you or your partner. Certain maternal high-risk medical conditions may also be potential causes of stillbirth. For example, those with diabetes mellitus, high blood pressure, or toxemia of pregnancy may be more predisposed to stillbirth because there is poor blood flow and nutrition to the fetus. In general, the cause of stillbirth in diabetics is less well understood. Other causes include IUGR, postmaturity, and umbilical accidents.

In other cases, the woman and fetus may be perfectly healthy when stillbirth occurs. One woman comments,

> We were really taken by surprise because my pregnancy was progressing so well. On Monday my obstetrician heard the baby's heart rate, and on Saturday I was told my baby had died inside of me three days earlier. The autopsy seemed to show that everything was normal, and the baby—we named him Pascal, was perfectly formed. My obstetrician was reluctant to give me a cause of the stillbirth, but after I pressed him he said that I may have had a virus or something that caused the baby to die.

Many couples are dissatisfied with the explanations given by health-care professionals, but, in many cases, professionals do not have all the answers. An autopsy may be done on your baby to give more clues about the death.

What to Expect

If this unfortunate event happens to you, you may no longer feel the fetus moving. One woman shares her experience:

> The week before my baby died, I had a feeling that something was not right. By the sixth month of pregnancy I was quite familiar with my baby's habits. I knew that the baby moved a great deal after I ate, but it had not done so for about one week. I also remarked that when I lay in bed on my side, it felt like my baby was very heavy on the side I was lying on, almost like dead weight, and certainly much heavier than she had been the week before. That's when I decided to go to the hospital.

Report any unusual occurrences to your physician. After trying to listen to your baby's heart rate with a stethoscope, an ultrasound will be done to assess your baby's well-being. The incidence of stillbirth is lower today, thanks to technological advances. Fetal monitors help detect the need for immediate interventions, such as a cesarean, when the baby's oxygen supply is diminished.

If your baby has died (there is no heartbeat), you will be given the difficult choice of choosing between immediate labor induction or waiting until labor begins on its own, which may take up to two weeks. If you choose induction, prostaglandins will be used. If you choose to wait for labor to begin naturally, the waiting may seem long, although some claim that it can give you and your partner time to work through your grief. When given the choice, most women choose to be induced within one to two days.

When you are told your baby has died, you may be in shock; it is normal to deny everything you hear. You may not remember all the details of what you are told. It is important to ask again later to ensure that you are adequately informed and prepared. No question is a stupid question, especially when it is your body and your baby that are concerned.

Please don't tell them
you never got to know me

It is I whose kicks you will always remember,
　　I who gave you heartburn that dragons would envy,
　　I who couldn't seem to tell time and got your days and nights
　　　　mixed up,
It is I who acknowledged your craving for peach ice cream by
　　knocking the cold bowl off your belly,
　　I who went shopping and helped you pick out the "perfect"
　　　　teddy bear for me,
　　I who liked to be cradled in your belly and rocked off to
　　　　dreamy slumber by the fire,
It is I who never had a doubt about your love,
It is I who was able to put a lifetime of joy into an instant.

Pat Schwiebert

Your Emotions

It is normal to have feelings of anger and emptiness following a stillbirth. For so many months you and your partner have organized your life around your child-to-be. The bonding that occurred will leave you with a sense of disorganization. You may be inclined to brood over what you might have done to save the child. There is no reason to feel guilty or to try to bear the blame for this mishap. There is nothing you could have done to change the situation. Chances are that you did all you could do, and that was to seek professional attention.

　　Mourning the loss of an unborn child is different from mourning the death of someone who has already lived. When we mourn for a deceased person we have actual memories to hold on to and to think about. With an unborn child, there are only the dreams and fantasies that have occupied your mind from the beginning of the pregnancy. It is important to express these dreams and to talk about your pregnancy. Talking may help you come to grips with your situation and assist you in getting back into your life.

　　Some mothers find that being able to hold their baby, even for a few minutes, helps them to acknowledge the loss. Taking a picture of the baby, taking footprints, saving the hospital bracelet, and giving the baby a name are also recommended. Some hospitals take routine photos and keep them on file, should the mother want to have them in the future. Seeing your baby right away may be difficult, but as time goes on you may regret not having that small yet sacred memory.

If you do decide to hold your baby, you should be aware that your baby may be different from your dreams and fantasies. Your baby will be cool to the touch and will be pale in color. Its skin may be peeling, and its head size may be smaller than expected. For some women, the thought of holding their dead baby is something they are unable to fathom. This is fine, too.

Many hospitals place mothers of stillborns in the maternity unit. It is difficult to be surrounded by women carrying their newborn bundles as you stroll the corridor empty-handed. This makes the grieving process much more difficult. If this is a problem for you, request early discharge from the hospital or a change of wards.

One woman who had a stillbirth comments,

> The year following the death of my baby was the hardest year of my life. Nobody seemed to understand what I was going through. They didn't understand that my baby was a real person to me and that I was very sad when it died. I felt very isolated and depressed. I found that friends were avoiding me. I remember one incident where I saw a childhood friend on the street who knew I lost my baby, and she turned around and walked the other way when she saw me. I understand that at times people don't know what to say—but this made it particularly hard on me at a time when I really needed love.

NEWBORN DEATH

Neonatal death is a death within the first four weeks after birth. The birth of a premature baby is most often associated with neonatal death because its systems are too immature to sustain life on its own. The baby's lungs may be unable to provide the needed oxygen, and its immune system may not be developed enough to fight infections. Severe congenital problems may also cause neonatal death because the nature of the abnormality is incompatible with life. These include problems associated with the heart, brain, kidneys, lungs, and/or endocrine system. Other possible reasons for neonatal death include those babies with Rh sensitization factors, those in fetal distress, those with chromosome abnormalities, and those with a combination of these factors.

After enduring labor or cesarean birth, the couple has already formed a bonding relationship with the new baby. The child may have had health problems that the couple has had to learn to accept. There may have already been some thoughts about the loss of the child. As the child goes through the crisis period, the parents experience a sense of uncertainty as they are torn between becoming more attached to the child and slowly distancing themselves in preparation for possible death. One husband explains,

> One of the hardest aspects of having our daughter in the premature nursery was the fact that although she was surrounded by excellent quality care she was also surrounded by death. There were so many infants so much sicker than she was— the sounds of emergency alarm systems beeping intermittently made me feel very ill at ease. We had already lost a baby from miscarriage and I couldn't bear losing another, especially one that I was already able to touch and hold.

In some cases the couple is aware of the possibility of death immediately following birth. The newborn may be in the high-risk unit being monitored very carefully. Twins are often at risk, and parents surviving the loss of one twin may have great difficulties coping. In most instances, when a couple experiences the death of a twin it is very difficult to grieve over the loss while rejoicing at the birth of the other baby. It is normal for the parents to have conflicting emotions as they try to retain enough strength and positive energy to give to the surviving child. Speaking with other parents who are in or were in similar situations can be very helpful. If you are comfortable in group situations, you should seek out a support group in your area. Or you may prefer the help of counselors specially trained in working with couples who have lost a baby or child.

In other cases, the death of a newborn is entirely unexpected. One woman explains,

Two years ago, our baby was born four weeks early and was doing extremely well. Although she was in the premature nursery, she was one of the healthiest newborns there. I was nursing her and she didn't have any tubes and wasn't hooked up to any machines. After having already had two miscarriages, I was sure that I was going to take this baby home. Well, I never did. Four days before I was to take her home, she developed what was to be a fatal staphylococcus infection. To this day, the shock I feel is overpowering.

Another woman was more poetic:

It felt like corn popping
Or maybe a wave
Surely there is a baby on the way.
The days will become fewer
Months of waiting will come to a close
Soft and pink with ten little toes.

The once empty spare room
Will now be filled with toys
Everything imaginable for our baby's joy.
But then something went wrong
Two months early the baby came
Quickly we had to think of a name.

We named our baby Brian
Brian meant "strong"
But he did not live very long.
We are thankful that we have Michael
And maybe soon another
Michael would love a sister or brother.

Debbie Schleigh

SUDDEN INFANT DEATH SYNDROME (SIDS)

Sudden infant death, sometimes called crib or cot death, is the unexpected death of an apparently healthy infant. In the United States, SIDS is responsible for approximately seven thousand to eight thousand deaths each year. In Canada, approximately 1,000 infants die from this syndrome each year. It is the leading cause of death in children one week to one year old. SIDS is not predictable or preventable, nor is it anyone's fault. It may happen to breast-fed or bottle-fed babies.

How it Happens

When and why SIDS happens remains an ongoing question for both parents and professionals. Typically, an infant is put to bed for the night or for its usual daytime nap with no suspicion of anything out of the ordinary. After some time, the child is found dead. Parents and caretakers have remarked that the baby does not seem to struggle, nor was there any crying or unusual sounds prior to death. The event is devastating.

Studies agree that the highest incidence of SIDS is between the ages of two and four months, with a peak at twelve weeks. The child often has a cold or other minor illness. It occurs most commonly in the winter months, although it may occur during any season.

The American Academy of Pediatrics now recommends that newborns be placed on their back or side while sleeping to help prevent SIDS. Since 1992, the year this recommendation was made, the rate of SIDS has dropped by 38 percent in the United States.

Causes of SIDS

Some infants are considered to be at high risk for SIDS, and professionals recommend that these infants have baby monitors in their room that ring when breathing ceases. Some professionals believe that the problem begins during prenatal development. An abnormal or underdeveloped respiratory system may prevent these infants from responding to carbon-dioxide levels in the blood that serve as the signal to breathe. As a result, they have periods of apnea (nonbreathing) even when they are awake.

Babies at Increased Risk for SIDS

○ Premature babies

○ Low-birth-weight babies

○ Twins and triplets

○ Children of smokers

○ Children of adolescent mothers

○ Children of mothers who did not receive adequate prenatal care

○ Children of methadone addicts

○ Children of low-income families

○ Children of mothers with high caffeine intake during pregnancy

○ Native Americans, African Americans

Remember, most of the babies who fall into one or more of these categories thrive and do very well. If your baby falls into any of these categories it does not mean that it will have the symptoms most commonly associated with SIDS but that the risk is greater than for the general population.

Many theories about the causes of SIDS have been proposed, including an allergy to cow's milk, viral infections, spinal hemorrhages, calcium/magnesium deficiency, excessive sodium (salt) in the blood, carbon dioxide pooling in the blood, heart/lung defects, house-mite allergy, stress, and lack of lung surfactant (a substance important in controlling surface tension in the lungs).

Coping with SIDS

Coping with the loss of a child to SIDS is very difficult because the situation is completely out of your control, and it may take a long time to resolve your feelings of helplessness. It is normal to feel guilty and angry, especially when it is difficult to identify the cause of your child's death. It is not uncommon for marriages to weaken after such an incident, or for fathers to immerse themselves in their work as their way of coping with the stress of losing a child. You may find that your husband is less communicative during this time and, like yourself, needs extra love and understanding.

Explaining what happened to other siblings may be a trying task, depending upon their ages. Younger children may not comprehend what has happened but may be sensitive to your moods and feelings of depression. They may need more love and affection and may use attention-seeking behaviors to get it. It may help if you can clarify or interpret your child's perception of what has happened. It is common for adults to deny that children are sad. Experiencing a loss can be a learning experience for a child—he or she can learn that the sadness is eventually resolved.

With younger children, try to be as simple as possible with your explanation. Mention that the baby died suddenly and unexpectedly, and that the baby seemed well and healthy when it died. They should be told that the death was nobody's fault. Older children may be told the facts about SIDS discussed above. Remember that children have different ways of coping with grief. They may become naughty, have nightmares, revert to bedwetting, or have other problems at school or at home.

Family, friends, and neighbors need to understand about SIDS. The popular misconceptions may make you uncomfortable when speaking with these people. Uninformed persons may believe that the baby was abused or neglected or suffocated in its bedding. These misconceptions and the negative attitudes associated with them make coping difficult. You may feel that you have nobody to talk to and that nobody understands what you are going through. If this is the case, you should seek professional help from someone who has experience with couples like yourselves. It is important that significant others understand that SIDS is not preventable, nor is it anyone's fault.

Future Pregnancies

The loss of a child to SIDS should not prevent you from becoming pregnant again. It is usually recommended that the mother not become pregnant until she has had an opportunity to deal with the loss of her baby. Having one SIDS baby does not necessarily lead to having another SIDS baby. Your pediatrician may carefully watch your baby after birth for any clues of respiratory difficulties. For the first year of your baby's life, it may be recommended that you use a monitor in your baby's room. Rather than being afraid,

you should be confident in knowing that you are doing everything in your power to ensure that it does not happen again.

THE GRIEVING PROCESS

Accepting your baby's death does not occur overnight, but rather
over weeks or months. It may take some women up to a year to
begin recovering from the deep pain of this tragedy. You may be
surprised at yourself for being so grief-stricken. What you are feeling is perfectly normal. Grieving is an important part of the
resolving process, and of accepting your loss so you can move on
with your life.

No two people react in the same way to the stress of the
death of a loved one. The way you cope may be similar to the way
you have coped with other stresses. Sharing your feelings with
others who have experienced loss can help you cope during this
difficult period. The Compassionate Friends is a group with over
five hundred chapters throughout the United States and over
thirty in Canada, plus chapters in other countries, whose goal is
to support and provide friendship and education for a bereaved
parent. One representative comments,

> Sharing and telling our stories over and over again is what
> the healing process is all about. We also learn that we are
> not "going crazy" and most of our feelings and the things we
> do or do not do after the death of our children are really nor-
> mal. Others tell us what it was like for them, too. We read
> books, listen to tapes, and listen to others who have suc-
> ceeded in resolving many of the problems and concerns of
> bereaved parents.

The loss of a child is a loss unlike any other. It is the loss of
something you have created. It is the loss of a loved one whom
you hardly knew, but knew very well. It is the loss of a special and
intense bond that was created over a very short period of time. In
a sense, when you lose a baby, you lose part of yourself.

When you lose a baby, there is deep disappointment, a loss of
hope and of plans for the future. Accepting this change in your
dreams and goals is not something that is accomplished

overnight. Your dreams are destroyed as you realize that the baby you grew to love is no longer there. One woman said that she was thankful to those who let her grieve:

> I'll never forget the emotional support I got from my closest friend. You really learn a great deal about people during these difficult times. It was especially surprising because she had never lost a baby, but she really knew me well. She was the only one who remembered the date of my child's death and one year later to the date sent me a card. It was nice to see that someone else also remembered my loss. Sometimes it's what people call "the little things" that really count.

Feelings of despair are common among those who lose a baby. These feelings are especially common in those who have had infertility problems or high-risk pregnancies. Where before all their energy and time centered around the new baby, now their life suddenly feels meaningless and empty. Borg and Lasker, in their book *When Pregnancy Fails*, state that feelings of despair may increase if the baby's sex was the one the parents had wished for. For example, if a family had three girls and wanted a boy and the boy died during delivery, the despair will be much more profound.

Everyone is affected differently following the loss of a loved one. The following are some of the most common reactions.

Physical Signs of Grieving

- Difficulty sleeping

- Bad dreams

- Loss of appetite

- Loss of energy

- Restlessness

- Muscle aches and pains

- Palpitations

- Stomach aches

- Diarrhea, constipation

Emotional Signs of Grieving

O Crying

O Apathy

O Irritability

O Uncontrollable sadness

O Confusion

O Indecision

O Feelings of going crazy

Very few people experience all these symptoms. You may have some, or none at all. But remember that they are normal expressions of the stress that you are going through.

Some women have identified grief as feeling as if they were locked in a dark closet without the key. You may feel that life is passing you by and you are just a spectator, unable to become involved. You may need someone, a dear friend or a professional, to help you get out of that closet. It is normal to have your ups and downs as you begin healing from your loss. You may take your problems out on others—this, too, is normal. It is a good idea to vent your concerns. Speaking with those who care is very important. One woman comments,

> Keep in the company of those who make you feel happy and good about yourself rather than those who tend to bring you down. It is important that you get on with your life while at the same time understanding that you should give yourself the necessary time to mourn.

The grieving parent cannot look to family and friends for understanding if they have not experienced the death of a child themselves. They will go back to their regular routines soon after the funeral, and we cannot count on them for the support we so need. Six months after the death, they expect us to be back to normal, and this is totally unrealistic. It is common for people to say, "Get on with your life and forget it." We do not want to forget our child. I feel that "to forget" means we could not have loved very much. We shall never "get over" the death, but we will learn to live with our grief, and the pain somehow becomes bearable.

SIGNIFICANT OTHERS

Fathers

Your partner will not be exempt from the grief-stricken reaction. You may think your grief is deeper because you were closer to the child, but chances are that he is hurting and is sheltering you from his pain. It is common for men to bond with the baby either later in pregnancy or after delivery, and therefore they tend to mourn the loss of a child differently than a woman. He may sublimate his pain by working long hours. If he was talkative before, he may become more quiet. It is not uncommon for the partner to block out the loss at first, and when the mother has begun to accept the loss a few months down the road, he may be starting to hurt.

You may be busy trying to resolve your own grief, and if you have other children your energy may need to be extended to them. Often the husband's needs are either neglected or overlooked. Although they too have experienced loss, men are still expected to continue making major decisions and to remain strong for their wives. Marriage failure and divorce are common following the death of a child. Studies have shown that divorce occurs in over 50 percent of those couples sustaining perinatal death, serious newborn abnormalities, and/or mental retardation. The spouses are unable to support one another because they are having difficulty supporting themselves through their own grief. It is common for one spouse to place blame on the other to cover up for their personal sense of failure. One woman comments,

> Losing our child was the most traumatic time in both our lives. Although we had known the child for such a short period of time, we felt a terrific void in our life. If it wasn't for local support groups for bereaved parents, I don't know what might have happened to either of us, or our relationship, for that matter.

Husbands often feel helpless, and as if they are "onlookers" during the pregnancy. When death occurs, they may feel even more alienated. It is important that both partners make an effort to give strength to one another. Couples should try to talk about the baby and about what their aspirations were.

The Sitting Time

Don't listen to the foolish unbelievers
    who say forget.
Take up your armful of roses and
    remember them
    the flower and the fragrance.
When you go home to do your sitting
    in the corner by the clock
    and sip your rosethorn tea.
It will warm your face and fingers
    and burn the bottom of your belly.
But as her gone-ness piles in white,
    crystal drifts,
It will be the blossom of her moment
    the warmth on your belly,
    the tiny fingers unfolding,
    the new face you've always known,
    that has changed you.
Take her moment, and hold it
    as every mother does.
She will always be
    your daughter.
And when the sitting is done you'll find
    bitter grief could never poison
    the sweetness of her time.

                                Joe Digman

Siblings

Siblings will grieve in their own way. Some may act inappropriately. The child senses the parents' tension and reacts to these feelings. It may be their first loss, and often they are unsure how to act, what to say, and how to grieve. If they are old enough, it is important to give them accurate and honest information about what has happened. Children also need to be told that they were not responsible for the loss and that guilt feelings are unnecessary. Try not to alienate them. Try to involve them in as many activities as possible. If they are older, there is no reason they cannot be a part of family discussions.

Younger children may have a more difficult time dealing with the death because they don't understand why it happened. They may be very fearful about what has occurred. They may also blame themselves for the death. Younger kids may have a fear of being abandoned following the death of a sibling, especially if they are under the age of five. Younger children may also surprise you with their reaction to the loss. As one woman says,

> Josh was two when his brother died. Although their relationship was short-lived, he seemed to be as grief-stricken as we were. His rapport with the baby began when I was pregnant, and how he enjoyed feeling and seeing the baby move inside of me. When the baby was born, he was very protective and loving to his younger brother. Now, two years after his death, he continues to ask questions about how and why his brother died. I find this amazing for a four-year-old. We decided to plant two trees in our backyard—one for each boy. Josh was very proud to help me do this. He tells everyone who the second tree was for—that was for my baby brother who died a long time ago, he says.

It is common for children to feel that wishing will bring the baby back, and it is important to explain to them that this will not happen. Tell them that most people live to be older before they die, but sometimes little babies and kids die because they are sick. Answer all their questions as simply as possible without overwhelming them.

FUTURE PREGNANCIES

Experiencing the loss of a baby should not prevent you from becoming pregnant again. Some women speak of another pregnancy even while they are in the hospital, with a sense of urgency to become pregnant again, while others fear the thought. It is important that you recover both physically and psychologically first. Many professionals recommend waiting anywhere from six months to one year before becoming pregnant again.

If you are over the age of thirty, you are probably battling time constraints and know that if you want to have a few children it is not a good idea to wait too long. Some women find it easier to have a child very soon after they lose a baby, while others are too afraid that the same thing will happen again. One woman who had one child and then a stillbirth said that she needed a break and was going to go back to school for a couple of years before deciding if she was going to have a second child.

It is normal to have fears and concerns with your subsequent pregnancy, but it is important not to let these emotions overwhelm you, because they could be detrimental to both you and your child-to-be. You may feel nervous and unsure of your situation. You may magnify each symptom and event and fear that they will result in the death of another baby. Remember, do not be hard on yourself or on others.

For the high-risk mother, having another baby is often a relief. It is common to have feelings of elation and appreciation for everything that goes right. Many women compare the new baby with the deceased one because the memories live on. But remember, this baby is a new one in its own right, with an identity of its own.

In some cases, another pregnancy may not be feasible because of your age or the complications of the earlier loss. The alternatives discussed in chapter 3 may be real possibilities for you. Perhaps adoption is your only option. The waiting is sometimes lengthy, but raising your child will be well worth the wait!

HELPFUL PUBLICATIONS

Understanding Grief When a Child Dies
Stillbirth, Miscarriage, and Infant Death
The Compassionate Friends, Inc.
P.O. Box 3696
Oak Brook, IL 60522-3696

Chapter 11

———————— O ————————

Cesarean Birth

The number of cesarean deliveries is on the rise. During the first two decades of this century, delivery by cesarean section (C-section) made up 1 to 3 percent of all deliveries. In the 1930s, when hospitals became the primary birthplace, the number began increasing. From the mid-1960s to the mid-1970s, the rate increased 12 to 20 percent annually. Current statistics indicate that the number may continue to rise. In North America, cesarean deliveries now account for approximately 21 percent of the 3.9 million babies born each year. In institutions specializing in high-risk pregnancies, the rate may go even higher.

Years ago cesareans were only performed when the life of the mother or the child was in serious jeopardy. Today, cesareans are not exclusively emergency procedures—they have become almost routine.

A midforceps delivery is sometimes, in some hospitals, used as an alternative to cesarean birth. Forceps are used during the second stage of labor to help the baby out if labor is prolonged, if the mother is exhausted, or if the baby shows signs of distress. Forceps delivery may, in rare instances, cause irreversible problems for the baby, such as cerebral palsy or learning difficulties. In most instances, there is less damage with a cesarean birth than with risking a difficult midforceps delivery. Low forceps deliveries are acceptable and safe, with a much lower risk of harm to the baby. For this reason, they are now more commonly used than midforceps.

Another, more frequently used alternative to cesarean is vacuum-assisted delivery. This is most often used when the baby's heartbeat slows or becomes erratic, when the baby's position makes delivery difficult, or when the mother is too tired to push.

The device used is a plastic or silicone cup applied to the baby's head and held in place by suction. Using a handle on the cup, the doctor is able to gently deliver the baby. Statistics show that the number of deaths and injuries from these devices is approximately 1 out of every 45,455 vacuum extractions per year.

WHY THE INCREASE

One reason for the increase in cesareans was the advent of the fetal monitor, which can accurately detect the health status of the fetus. It has been in use since the 1970s and is an invaluable tool in identifying fetal distress through monitoring of the baby's heart rate.

There has been controversy surrounding the increased number of cesareans. Although not well supported, one theory is that making money is at the heart of the medical profession, and that to compensate for a decline in birth rates and a glut of obstetricians, more income-producing cesareans are carried out.

Some say that the reason for the increase is related to physicians' desire to minimize their risks, especially in light of the recent increase in malpractice suits. The "gray areas" of obstetrics, where the safety of vaginal birth may be questioned, may automatically result in a preventive cesarean birth in order to avoid known potential risks.

Despite these criticisms, the increase in cesarean births does have a positive side. Because of the high success rate, more children are born alive and healthy. There has been a definite decrease in fetal mortality and a significant decrease in infant deaths.

REASONS FOR A CESAREAN

Below is a summary of the most common indications for cesarean birth.

O Repeat cesarean due to previous surgery on the uterus

O Placenta previa, to prevent excessive maternal bleeding that may affect the fetus

O Abruptio placenta, to prevent rapid blood and oxygen loss to the baby as a result of the placenta separating

O Herpes infection, to prevent passing it on to the baby through the birth canal

O Severe toxemia, to prevent fetal complications

O Fetal distress as identified through ultrasounds and/or fetal monitoring

O Abnormal fetal position, such as breech or transverse presentation, making it impossible for the baby to pass through the birth canal

O Diabetic mother, if the disease results in a very large baby or poor blood flow to the placenta

O Prolapsed cord, to prevent loss of oxygen to the baby

O Cephalopelvic disproportion (CPD), if the baby's head is too large to pass through the birth canal

O Failure of labor to progress or if oxytocin has not been effective

O Forcep or vacuum failure

EMERGENCY CESAREANS

Whether you are a high-risk mother or not, it is a good idea to be prepared for the possibility of having a cesarean, because surprises do occur. Emergency cesareans are done only after a definitive diagnosis is made. A woman will have an emergency cesarean if there is pelvic disproportion (the baby is too big to fit through the birth canal), fetal distress (e.g., due to the umbilical cord wrapping around the fetus's neck, placental insufficiency, low oxygen, or infection), maternal distress, such as abruptio placenta, maternal heart problems, or toxemia of pregnancy. Although time will be of the essence, it is important that you ask for even a brief explanation for the surgery. It is also your prerogative to request a second opinion.

One second-time mother talks about how easy her first delivery was and how her second was high-risk right from the beginning:

In addition to being diagnosed as having gestational diabetes, my baby was in distress when I was in labor. I was on the fetal monitor, and after twelve hours of labor, meconium was found in the amniotic fluid, and my baby's heart rate dropped whenever I had a contraction. Changing positions did not alter his status. The fact that my baby's cord was around his neck made my entire delivery an emergency situation. Before I knew it I was being shaved for a cesarean. I just was not prepared for it. No one ever mentioned the chances of me having a cesarean, especially since the labor with my daughter went so well.

RISKS OF CESAREANS

Cesareans are much safer now than they were in the past. Today there is a better understanding of anesthesia and of postoperative recovery. The scars are smaller and they heal faster. The percentage of women who have complications as a result of cesarean delivery is low in comparison to the number of healthy mothers and babies undergoing the procedure. You should be aware of some possible complications, including infection, peritonitis (an inflammation of the membrane covering the abdominal wall), urinary-tract infection, and side effects from anesthesia. Pneumonia and thromboembolism (a blocked blood vessel due to a blood clot) are other problems that rarely occur today thanks to early mobilization following surgery and the increased number of cesareans performed under epidural anesthesia instead of general anesthesia.

Hemorrhage from a cesarean is rare today, but it is a risk that accompanies any operation. The uterus has numerous blood vessels and is particularly susceptible to hemorrhage. In the past, hemorrhage was often fatal. In large hospital centers today, hemorrhage is usually effectively treated with medications and intravenous therapy. The chance of uterine hemorrhage is one of the major reasons home deliveries are not recommended.

REPEAT CESAREANS

Having had a cesarean once does not necessarily mean you will always have to have a cesarean. The need for subsequent cesareans will depend upon the reason for the first one. If, for example, you had a cesarean because of a small pelvis, chances are that your second pregnancy will also result in a cesarean. If you had a cesarean because your baby was in a breech position and your second baby is not, then you may be able to have a normal vaginal delivery. The American College of Obstetricians and Gynecologists (ACOG) estimates that one in three of all cesareans are repeat cesareans.

Some physicians allow a trial vaginal labor following a cesarean, but often this remains a matter of professional judgment. Others may opt for repeat cesarean births because of the risk during prolonged labor of a ruptured uterus on the old incision. However, the risk of these problems is very low during trial labor—between 0.5 and 1.5 percent for women who have had a previous low transverse incision. Trial labor is a personal and professional decision to be made by the physician and the woman. You should discuss it early in your pregnancy.

In 1998, ACOG developed guidelines for vaginal delivery after a cesarean. Some of the conditions they recommend for considering a trial vaginal labor include the following:

◯ Women who have had a low transverse (bikini) incision from previous cesareans

◯ Women with a clinically adequate pelvis (size)

◯ Women who want a normal labor and delivery

◯ Women with no other uterine scars or previous rupture

◯ A physician readily available throughout labor capable of monitoring labor and performing an emergency cesarean delivery

◯ The availability of anesthesia and personnel for emergency cesarean delivery

◯ The availability of a physician who is capable of evaluating labor and performing a cesarean

It is a good idea to discuss the possibility of a vaginal birth after cesarean (VBAC) with your physician early in pregnancy. You should make your desires known, and he or she should share a similar philosophy. Keep in mind, however, that there is a chance you will have to have an emergency cesarean. It is estimated that 60 to 80 percent of VBACs result in successful vaginal births. The advantages include decreased chance of needing a blood transfusion, fewer infections, easier recovery, and no increased overall risk to the baby.

Here are some questions to ask your physician:

○ What are your feelings toward VBAC?

○ What are my chances of having a VBAC?

○ Will you permit me to have a trial labor? If no, why not?

○ What percentage of your patients have a successful VBAC?

BEFORE YOUR CESAREAN

Surgery is scary. No two people handle surgery or recuperation the same way, so what is suggested here should not be considered gospel. Any questions should be directed to your health-care team.

Presurgical Tests

If your cesarean is prearranged, you will most likely be admitted to the hospital the morning of your surgery. In most hospitals you will be admitted to the unit that you will be in after your baby is born—the postpartum unit. Request the same room after delivery. Some women prefer private rooms, while others prefer not to be alone. Some first-time mothers find it interesting talking with other mothers and sharing experiences. Others may feel that having a baby is a very private affair and may prefer to be alone with their baby and family during visiting hours.

Meeting the Anesthesiologist

The anesthesiologist, the person who helps make delivery less painful, will also want to meet with you before surgery. You will be asked some questions about your medical history, including your previous experiences with anesthesia.

The Shave

Before your cesarean, you may have to face having part of your pubic and abdominal area shaved. Years ago physicians requested that women have their entire pubic area shaved. Fortunately, today shaving is not an ordeal. The total area that is shaved, however, depends on your physician's personal preference and the institution's surgical protocol. Some physicians request that the woman lie on her bed with her legs together and have shaved whatever pubic hair is showing. Others still request complete pubic shaving, while a smaller number may allow the woman not to be shaved at all.

What—No Food?

The evening prior to your scheduled cesarean you will be told not to eat or drink anything after midnight. This is to avoid the possibility of regurgitating and aspirating the contents of your stomach during surgery. The nurses may hang a sign outside your room or above your bed which says "N.P.O." Do not worry, it is not a secret code among the staff—it stands for *non per os* (Latin for "not by mouth"). This is to remind the staff not to leave you drinks or food.

Intravenous Therapy

Some hospitals have a policy to insert an intravenous solution the night before or the morning of surgery. The solution is usually placed in a vein in your lower arm. Request that it not be put in the arm that you write with. This fluid is usually sugar water, or saline water if you are a diabetic. The solution will nourish you in the absence of food. If your mouth gets dry, ask your nurse for glycerine or lemon swabs to help lubricate and freshen your mouth. Ice chips are not usually allowed. The anesthesiologist may insert another intravenous drip in your arm when you are in the operating room. This will be used in case you need additional medication during surgery.

The Explanation

Before your cesarean, your nurse or physician should explain to you just what to expect. Both have probably explained the procedure many times before, so do not be shy to ask questions. It is your body, and you have a right to know. Make sure you get their name in case you have a question after they leave. Keep a pad and paper by your bed to write down questions that come to mind. One woman said that she never had questions during the explanation of the surgery. She remarks,

> My questions always arose late at night when the lights were off and I was trying to fall asleep. Reaching over to the bedside table to my pad saved me the agony of trying to remember the questions the following morning.

The Morning of Your Cesarean

On the morning of your cesarean, your nurse will ask you a few questions, such as

- O When did you drink last?
- O When did you last urinate?
- O Did you sign your consent form?
- O Does your family know you are going to have a cesarean? Where can they be reached?
- O Do you have any valuable items that you want to check at the nursing station?

You will also be asked if you are wearing contact lenses or nail polish or have any artificial parts, such as dentures. All artificial parts and nail polish must be removed. The operating room staff must be able to see the natural color of your nails to ensure that you have adequate blood flow. If you have ever seen cold, poorly oxygenated hands, you know how blue they can become!

THE TYPE OF ANESTHESIA

The type of anesthesia that is chosen depends upon the hospital's policies and your preference. General anesthesia puts a person completely to sleep. It is not used during labor because it slows down the entire process. Epidurals and spinal anesthesia are used in cesarean delivery. They provide numbness in the lower half of the body but allow a person to remain awake. Regional anesthesia is sometimes used in delivery, but not in cesareans.

Epidurals

Epidurals are given through a tiny catheter or tube placed in the back by a needle. An injection is made in the middle of the back and the catheter is moved into the epidural space, the space around the spinal column. The anesthetic is dripped in in carefully measured doses. Epidurals numb the area immediately around the perineum and lower uterus, belly to toes. They take between five and thirty minutes to be effective. When your legs feel warm, this is usually the first sign that this block is working. It usually remains effective for forty-five to sixty minutes. During your surgery, the anesthesiologist may add more through the tubing that remains in your lower back.

Epidurals can be useful when a woman has a serious respiratory disease, as the drug reduces the workload of the lungs. It is also used for diabetics, as it reduces the demands on the body's metabolism. It is used increasingly for cesarean sections.

Spinal Anesthesia

Spinal anesthesia is used during delivery to anesthetize the entire birth area (from belly to toes). The anesthesiologist injects spinals into the subarachnoid space around the spinal column. Spinals stop labor and the ability to bear down. Some aftereffects include headache, stiff neck, and backache. You will need to remain flat on your back for a period of time following delivery because postspinal headache is possible. Spinals are frequently given for cesarean delivery.

General Anesthesia

General anesthesia is usually used in emergency C-sections or in unusual situations. It is preferred that you not eat for six to eight hours prior to anesthesia; however, in an emergency, these guide-lines may be modified. Studies have shown that babies born to mothers who have general anesthesia tend to be temporarily lethargic after birth and do not respond as quickly as babies born under epidurals. However, being asleep during an operation has its positive side, as you do not hear or see what is going on around you. For some, the sounds of the operating room and the talk of the staff may be frightening and threatening.

Epidurals/Spinals vs. General Anesthesia

Epidurals and spinals are generally quite safe and may have many advantages over general anesthesia. Being awake for the birth of a baby, one of the most exciting moments in a woman's life, is obviously desirable. Another advantage is that in most modern teaching institutions your husband is allowed to be with you. For some women, this is a very important consideration. It is incred-ible how he can make a difference by comforting you and hold-ing your hand. If your husband accompanies you into the operat-ing room, he will usually be seated next to you near your head. There is usually a drape that conceals your lower body so that neither you nor your husband sees the actual surgery, though some eager husbands may stand up on their toes to see the birth of the baby on the other side of the curtain.

Many institutions do not allow spouses into the operating room if a woman is under general anesthesia; however, you should ask the staff if it is possible. If this is not allowed, see if your part-ner can view the baby as soon after the birth as possible—this will probably be long before you are awake.

THE SURGERY

Cesareans must be performed in hospitals with adequate supplies, drugs, anesthesia, antibiotics, and blood transfusion equipment. After being washed and swabbed with a special antiseptic solution, your lower abdomen will be covered with surgical "drapes" or cloths. The only area that is exposed is the area where the incision will be.

You will receive your anesthesia, and when your abdomen is numb or when you are unconscious, the obstetrician will make a small horizontal cut in your abdominal wall, down near your pubic hairline. Vertical incisions are done less frequently today, though in a severe emergency they may be done to remove the baby more quickly.

A cut is then made horizontally in the uterine muscle and the baby is eased out. If you are awake, this is an amazing moment. It is exciting hearing the first cry. The nurses will immediately suction your baby's nose and mouth with a fine mucus catheter. When the baby is breathing well, you or your partner will be able to hold your child. While you are holding your baby, the physician removes the placenta and you are sewn back together, layer by layer. You will then be transferred to the recovery room.

AFTER YOUR CESAREAN

If the cesarean is your first surgery, it might be frightening. It is a strange sensation to know that your skin was cut and your insides exposed. If your cesarean is done under emergency circumstances and you were prepared with prenatal classes, you may feel that all those hours of deep breathing and panting went down the drain. You may also feel a sense of disappointment and depression because you were unable to have a vaginal delivery. Some women find it very difficult to adapt to having given birth by cesarean and want to speak with other women who have had similar experiences. Local support groups can be sought out by speaking with the hospital's social worker or the nurses in your postpartum unit. For other women, these feelings of disappointment are less, especially if getting pregnant was a problem.

Your Incision

One of the primary concerns of many people having surgery is the appearance of their incision. Today, cesarean incisions are smaller and less noticeable than they were years ago. More often than not, the incision is low, and is sometimes called a "bikini incision." As its name implies, you will be able to wear a bikini afterward without your scar showing.

The other type of incision runs vertically on the abdomen. This incision is rarely used today. It is chosen only if the placenta is in an unusual position, if the delivery is very premature, if time

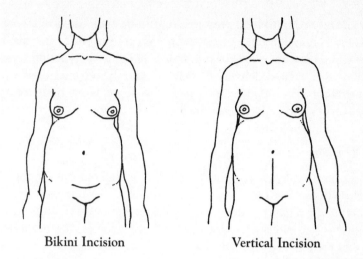

Bikini Incision   **Vertical Incision**

is an important factor, or if you have had a previous midline vertical incision.

The preparation for the surgery and the suturing of your incision will take more time than the birth itself. It may take only five to ten minutes from the time the incision is made for your baby to be born and about forty-five minutes to suture the six or seven layers of incisions. The only sutures that are visible are those on the outer layer. Today, surgical staples are most commonly used, though some centers may also use clamps and/or other adhesives.

The Recovery Room

Depending upon the institution, you will be transferred to a recovery room when your baby goes to the nursery. In most centers the babies are brought to the mother as soon as she is in the recovery room—usually within one hour after birth. The La Leche League, for example, strongly advocates nursing as soon as possible after delivery. In some cases, if the woman is unable to hold her baby immediately, the husband can be given the chance to get involved with the baby's immediate care. Many husbands feel great rewards from becoming involved.

In the recovery room or intensive care unit, the nurses will carefully monitor your vital signs, such as heart rate, breathing, temperature, and blood pressure. Your nurse will also check your lochia (vaginal discharge). Some women are surprised how much bleeding they have after a cesarean, although it is sometimes less than with vaginal delivery. It may be quite heavy after delivery, saturating about two to four pads. By about eight hours after delivery it will be like a normal menstrual flow.

The Exam

Your uterus may be very tender when touched, but the examination will not last long. The nurse will check to see if your uterus is contracting and returning to its original size. Oxytocin/syntocinon is sometimes given intravenously to help your uterus return to its predelivery size. If it does not do so, this may be a sign of excessive bleeding.

The Catheter

Prior to going to the operating room, a urinary catheter will have been inserted to monitor your urine output. This usually remains in place for anywhere from six to thirty-six hours after your cesarean, depending on both your physician and how you are doing. Initially the catheter is uncomfortable, and then it becomes more of a nuisance than anything else. You should know that it is necessary.

After the catheter is removed it may sting when you pass urine the first time, so try not to be alarmed. Some women say that it feels like a needle is being inserted in them. This feeling does not last long.

When Does the Anesthesia Wear Off?

If you had general anesthesia, you will probably sleep for a few hours in the recovery room after your baby is born. If you had an epidural, you will be awake but most likely drowsy. With epidurals you are usually allowed to return to the postpartum unit when you are able to move your legs. They may seem numb and clumsy at first, but this is the first sign of the anesthesia wearing off. It is usually possible to move your legs about two hours after delivery, but this varies.

Deep Breathing and Coughing

Very soon after your cesarean you will be told of the importance of deep breathing and coughing. This is especially important for a woman who has had general anesthesia. After you lie in one position without moving for several hours, secretions tend to accumulate in your lungs. Stagnant secretions are an ideal haven for bacterial growth, such as that which causes pneumonia. "Huffing" is another way to loosen secretions in the lungs and may be more comfortable for you. Try exhaling forcefully through your mouth. Support your incision with your hand or a pillow during deep breathing and coughing exercises. Huffing should also make these important exercises more comfortable for you after your cesarean and in the weeks that follow. Deep breathing and coughing, walking, and drinking plenty of fluids are invaluable to help loosen unwanted secretions.

Pain

While in the recovery room, you will be given intravenous pain relievers. You may have two intravenous lines, one inserted before your cesarean and another one inserted by the anesthesiologist in the operating room. One is usually removed in the recovery room, the other a few days later when you are drinking and eating well. If your incision hurts, do not be shy about asking your nurse for a pain reliever.

Very soon after your anesthesia wears off, you will start to feel your incision. It seems that every move you make is the wrong one. Some women have difficulty finding a comfortable position, and it may be very tempting to not move at all—but do not do that because it may increase your problems later. The most uncomfortable times are getting in and out of bed, and when you are doing your deep breathing and coughing exercises.

One recent advance has been the use of patient-controlled analgesia (PCA). Basically, this is a pump from which the new mother can self-administer pain medication intravenously as needed. Prior to having your cesarean, you will be told how to use this device. It is usually only needed for twenty-four hours following the delivery.

Eating and Drinking

Eating and drinking are not allowed until bowel function resumes, usually later in the day after delivery. Your abdomen will be examined with a stethoscope for sounds of bowel function. If sounds are heard, you will be able to drink and later to eat. Make sure to ask for glycerine swabs to relieve mouth dryness. Some hospitals will provide ice chips. Your first meal will be very light food—tea, clear broth, and/or Jell-O.

Gas Pains

Gas pains are very common following cesarean birth because your bowel was manipulated during surgery in order to expose your uterus. Gas pains are usually worst on the third day after the cesarean, the time when bowel function returns to normal.

To relieve or reduce gas pains, lie on your left side and draw your knees against your chest; try breathing with your abdomen; try getting up and walking around; ask the nurse to massage your upper abdomen from right to left; avoid fruit juices and drinking through straws.

One woman comments on gas pains:

They warned me about gas pains following my cesarean. They also told me that I should avoid gas-producing foods and carbonated beverages. It's funny, because one of the things that I found most soothing for my gas pains was ginger ale—I don't know if it was the ginger or the carbonation that was so soothing. All I know is that I drank an awful lot of it with great relief.

Getting Out of Bed

Most hospital units allow you to get out of bed after the anesthesia has completely worn off—about six or eight hours later. You may feel very uncomfortable when you try this for the first time. Two helpful tips are to ask for your pain reliever about half an hour before you get out of bed, and walk a little farther each time. Remember, the more you lie still, the stiffer you become and the more uncomfortable it will be for you when you eventually start to move about.

Everyone heals at a different rate. You may feel wonderful one day and lousy the next. This is normal. Many women say that the third day after surgery is the most difficult; this is usually when the healing process begins. There are usually great improvements, however, the following day.

Rooming-In

The decision whether to room-in—have your baby sleep in your room during the night—is entirely up to you. Some mothers feel that once they get home they will not have a choice whether or not they look after their baby. They therefore choose to get as much rest as possible in the hospital, and allow the night nurses to feed the baby. Rest, although sometimes difficult for a new mother, is very important, especially for the mother who has had a cesarean. Some mothers choose to room-in from the third day onward, while others choose to room-in just the evening before discharge.

BREAST-FEEDING AFTER A CESAREAN

Whatever type of feeding method you choose, the fact that you had a cesarean should not interfere with your plans. Until recently, many hospitals did not permit immediate breast-feeding following cesarean delivery. Ask if immediate breast-feeding is possible in your institution. If not, you should be consoled by knowing that if the baby is born strong and healthy, it will be fine for the first six hours of life without any food. By then you should be feeling stronger and be in your bed in the postpartum unit. You can ask your nurse to bring your baby so you can breast-feed. If you are not up to it, do not feel guilty if you delay this first feeding.

I remember feeling happy when I was told that my baby would not require feeding for six hours but that I would be able to nurse her after that. I wanted to establish the infant-mother bond that we hear so much about and was glad that the cesarean did not get in our way. Those six hours gave me a chance to recover from the surgery and gave her a chance to get used to life on her own.

Positioning

Finding a comfortable nursing position is often a challenge following a cesarean delivery. It is normal to feel clumsy at first. You must find the position that is right for you. Many women find lying in bed very uncomfortable and prefer to be seated in a chair with a pillow on their lap and the baby on top of the pillow. Others find holding the baby in a football hold with the baby's head cupped in their hand and feet directed toward their back, away from the abdomen, to be a comfortable position. Lying on your side may also be comfortable. Choosing a good breast-feeding position is a very personal decision.

In most cases you will be able to continue taking your pain relievers while breast-feeding, although some babies may become a bit drowsy as a result. If you need pain relievers, remind the hospital staff that you are nursing. Advil or Tylenol are good choices that won't interfere with breast-feeding and should not make you drowsy.

RECOVERY

Your recovery from a cesarean will depend upon your individual recuperative powers, the type of anesthesia you had, and the length of time you were in labor prior to your cesarean. One first-time mother who had general anesthesia said,

> I felt so wiped out for so many days afterward that it took me a long time to get my feet on the ground. At the birth of my second child, I had an epidural, and, gee, what a world of difference! I was up and about that same evening. I felt alive and ready to begin mothering. If given a choice, I think all mothers should choose an epidural over general anesthesia. I didn't feel like I was hit over the head with a baseball bat.

Regardless of the type of anesthesia, the most difficult part about a cesarean is the recovery. Do not expect to go bouncing down the hall the same evening and be sitting in the lounge chatting with other mothers for hours on end. Avoid bringing stacks of books or knitting to the hospital, and do not plan on getting back to your daily swimming routine when you get home. Plan on being just a little more tired and maybe a little more irritable. It's all normal! And remember the most important thing— it only gets better!

GOING HOME

Today, hospitalization for cesareans is usually about three days. Do not expect to be able to do too much right away at home. Your incision will be tender and you will be regaining your strength.

One mother who had twins by a cesarean remarks,

> I had to learn to let the house go. I had the twins plus one twenty-month-old in diapers. My bed was unmade for the first six months. I actually spent the first month in the lazy chair with one twin breast-feeding and the other one at my feet. You just really have to take it in stride.

Lifting

You will not be able to lift anything heavy for the first six weeks after your cesarean. If everything goes well, the usual recommended weight is under ten pounds, and if you are lucky that should include your baby! Try bending your knees when lifting your baby; this helps your legs do the lifting rather than your back or your abdomen. You'll have more of a problem if there are other children at home. Your toddler may not understand why you can lift the baby and not him or her. He or she may show signs of regression. If you were unable to lift your children during the pregnancy because of complications, there will not be much of a change. If you were able to lift them, you might have your hands full—emotionally and physically. The best advice is to be patient and to try to get the toddler involved in the care of the new baby as much as possible. Ask him or her to do things like going to get a diaper or bringing the baby a toy. Like all of us, children love to feel needed.

If you can arrange to have help for the first few weeks, all the better. Some husbands choose to take their vacation at this time, and it is a lovely way for the baby to start its first few weeks of life. One mother of a two-and-a-half-year-old came home to the same responsibilities she left behind. Her husband worked long, hard hours, and not only did she not have any family or professional help, but she had a toddler, a baby, and a cesarean to contend with. She comments,

> People really don't understand what a cesarean birth involves. Mine was an emergency one and I was so naïve. I had no idea it would be like this. My attitude has changed now. Who cares if my house is messy or the laundry is not done? It is not humanly possible to do it all—my priorities have changed under the circumstances.

Stairs

If there are stairs leading to your bedroom, you will soon learn that they present a problem. If you have had a vertical incision, it is recommended that you not climb stairs for one to two weeks. With a bikini incision, you can gradually do the stairs with assistance, taking one step at a time. Try slowly increasing your activity. Start going up and down once a day, then twice a day, and so on. The best advice is to see how you feel. If you have excruciating pain after activity, you were probably trying to do too much. Listen to your body—it will give you all kinds of signals. Do not forget to ask your caregiver what is recommended.

Walks

If you have your baby during warm weather, going out for walks can be very refreshing for both you and the baby. It will be a few weeks before you will be able to push a stroller, but you should make a habit of getting out each day. Mentally and physically, it is healthy for both of you. Try walking a little bit farther each day.

It takes about six weeks to recover fully from a cesarean. After that time your incision is completely healed and you can safely lift heavier objects. The six weeks pass very quickly, and before you know it you are well on your way to getting back into your normal routine—if there is such a thing for today's mother!

HELPFUL PUBLICATIONS

The VBAC Companion: The Expectant Mother's Guide to Vaginal Birth After Cesarean by Diana Korte
Harvard Common Press
535 Albany Street
Boston, MA 02118
(800) 462-6240

Chapter 12

──────── O ────────

Premature Babies

For those who have had a normal pregnancy, a premature baby may be an entirely unexpected event. For the high-risk mother, however, having a premature baby ("preemie") may have been a foreseen possibility from the beginning.

The experience of having a premature baby is not easy, whether you are prepared or not. Sometimes women find it difficult juggling their own needs, their baby's needs, and their family's needs. There may be sudden feelings of overwhelming responsibility and helplessness. These are all normal. The background information and tips on coping with a preemie offered in this chapter should take some of the mystery out of one of life's most intense moments.

WHAT IS A PREMATURE BABY?

A premature or preterm baby is one born prior to the thirty-seventh completed week of gestation. According to the National Center for Health Statistics, 423,107 premature babies were born in 1996, accounting for approximately 11 percent of all births.

A small-for-gestational-age (SGA) baby is one that is smaller than average for its age. Unlike premature babies, SGA babies are well formed and usually have fully developed internal systems, although there are often complications due to their small size. Your baby's gestational age is figured by counting the number of weeks from the date of your last menstrual period. This simply refers to the amount of time, from conception to birth, that the baby spent in the womb.

CAUSES OF PREMATURITY

It is not always possible to identify the cause of a premature birth. Approximately 50 percent of premature births are due to unknown reasons. There are, however, certain high-risk situations that may render you more susceptible to having a premature baby.

Multiple gestation is a common cause of premature labor, primarily because the uterus becomes overly distended and goes into labor. Approximately half of all multiple pregnancies end in preterm delivery.

Incompetent cervix, which is a painless dilation of the cervix, will result in preterm delivery, sometimes in the second trimester. No contractions occur. Some daughters of women who took DES (diethylstilbestrol) during the 1940s and 1950s to prevent miscarriages are at risk of having been born with an incompetent cervix. Having had repeated D&Cs or having a septate uterus may also be a risk factor, although the reasons for this are not understood. Similarly, infections of the cervix or vagina can increase the risk.

Toxemia may be a cause of prematurity if the physician had to prematurely induce labor to resolve complications due to preeclampsia.

Placental problems, such as placenta previa and abruptio placenta, and excessive amniotic fluid (polyhydramnios) may also result in preterm delivery. Placenta previa, however, does not always result in preterm labor.

Certain environmental factors, such as insufficient diet, a history of excessive smoking, cocaine use, fetal alcohol syndrome (FAS), or fetal alcohol effect (FAE), may also result in your baby's early birth. Following an unsupervised weight-loss regime is never recommended during pregnancy. Women who are underweight or who weigh less than one hundred pounds are at risk. Alcoholic women often give birth to SGA infants, who may also be premature. Alcoholic women often have a poor diet; the direct consequences are fetal malnutrition and inadequate growth patterns. Women who receive little or no prenatal care may experience premature labor because of various untended complications.

Sometimes the cause of prematurity is not so easy to iden-tify. There simply may not be any more room inside the uterus for the baby to grow. Sometimes the baby is just ready to be born and your waters break. This is what happened to me during my first pregnancy.

The circumstances surrounding my preterm labor were very unusual. I was thirty-two weeks pregnant on the day of our sixth wedding anniversary. My husband felt that I had been through a lot during my pregnancy—seven months in bed, and many stressful moments. Since my baby had been viable at twenty-eight weeks, we felt that the real danger period was over, and he decided to take me to a very elegant resort for the night. The car trip involved two hours on a bumpy road. I cannot help but believe that the bumps stirred up something inside me, although my obstetrician did not really believe this was the cause of my preterm labor the following evening.

Your baby's early arrival may be due to a combination of fac-tors. It is normal to feel guilty and to ask yourself whether you did too much or if you did the wrong thing. Often what you imagine is worse than reality, so it is best to discuss your concerns with the professionals.

THE WARNING SIGNS

Ruptured membrane (breaking your water) occurs in approxi-mately 20 percent of women experiencing premature labor. The most common signs and symptoms include a feeling of pressure and/or a thin mucus or blood discharge. However, premature labor is not always accompanied by warning signs. Many women are unsure that they are having a preterm birth, mainly because the symptoms are not as obvious. Some women notice a dull ache in their lower back and unusual sensations in their abdomen without experiencing any labor pains. You may find that you have mild abdominal discomfort similar to menstrual cramps. These may or may not be accompanied by abdominal pressure and diarrhea. If you have these symptoms or experience four to six Braxton Hicks contractions (painless contractions) in one hour that don't stop after rest, contact your physician.

Bleeding may occur as a result of abruptio placenta or placenta previa. In the former, the bleeding is due to the separation of the placenta from the uterus, which immediately deprives the baby of essential nutrients and oxygen. A cesarean may then be necessary.

Women at risk for preterm delivery may consider a new option, the use of home uterine activity monitoring (HUAM). HUAM is a monitoring device worn on the abdomen twice a day for one hour. This device measures the frequency, duration, and intensity of contractions too faint for a woman to recognize on her own. The results may be transmitted digitally over the phone to a nurse or other specialist who can determine the next course of action.

At the hospital, you will be monitored for contractions and your cervix will be checked for dilation. Your baby's health will be evaluated using the electronic fetal monitor. Intravenous fluids or medications may be given to stop the contractions. It is possible that you will be sent home with medication and/or guidelines for restricted activity. In this case, you will need to monitor your contractions at home. Most women are allowed to stop taking medication and resume activity at thirty-six weeks.

CHARACTERISTICS OF PREMATURITY

Obviously, the premature baby is at higher risk than the full-term baby. What types of problems your baby has depends upon how premature it is and how advanced it is in its development. Most professionals will try to keep the baby inside of you as long as possible without risking your life or your baby's life. Your baby will mature better there than anywhere else—you are the best incubator.

Remember that each baby reacts differently to the stress of being born too early. Most important, remember that each baby has its own set of problems. Be fair to yourself and your baby, and do not attempt to compare your baby to the baby in the next crib.

Appearance

Physically, the premature baby looks different from the full-term baby. Some have described the preemie as looking like a frog, a rat, or even a chicken. The baby's skin will be very wrinkled, like that of an old person. Your baby's head will seem large in proportion to the rest of its body, and its arms and legs will be mere slender additions to a tiny body. Because premature babies have very little fat on their bodies, they become cold and blue (cyanotic) very quickly. For this reason, you will notice that bathing and diaper changes often need to be done fast.

Preemies are also relatively inactive and may appear limp at times. This may be nature's way of conserving their energy for growing. In general, they sleep more in the early stages of life—sleeping is as important as eating for them. It is also common for preemies to be both restless and somewhat irritable. Your baby will probably respond when it hears your voice and sees you in front of it. Speaking and cuddling are very important at this time.

Your baby's needs are similar to yours. It needs to breathe, be warm, eat, drink, urinate, have bowel movements, and be loved. Any interruption or interference with any of these needs may present a problem for your little one.

Breathing

Because its lungs and respiratory muscles are not adequately developed, your baby may have difficulty breathing on its own. Production of surfactant, the chemical that reduces the surface tension within the lungs, is necessary for the baby to expand its lungs and breathe on its own. Under normal circumstances, the fetus produces this chemical by the twenty-eighth week of gestation, but only in sufficient quantities by the thirty-fourth or thirty-fifth week. If premature delivery is anticipated, during pregnancy you may be given several doses of betamethasone, a corticosteroid that promotes your baby's lung maturity.

There is a newer form of therapy given after birth to promote lung maturity and prevent respiratory distress syndrome (RDS). It is the administration of the surfactant that the baby is unable to make, which, in the form of a fine mist, is put into the baby's oxygen mixture by mask or respirator. As the infant breathes, this mist enters the lungs.

Irregular breathing is common among preemies. You may notice that your baby takes many short breaths, then a long breath, and then rests for a few seconds. Although this may be scary for you, as your baby's lungs mature it will outgrow this type of breathing pattern. In the hospital the staff will carefully monitor the baby's breathing patterns by observing its chest movements and counting the number of breaths per minute. Hospital staff will also detect whether your baby's breathing pattern is regular, labored, deep, or shallow. A special monitor may be used to identify a change of pattern in your baby's breathing.

Respiratory Distress Syndrome (RDS)

RDS sometimes occurs when a baby is born unexpectedly and surfactant has not yet been produced. Without surfactant, the baby's lungs are unable to expand fully. This syndrome is successfully treated with oxygen therapy, humidity, and sometimes medications. A special machine called CPAP (continuous positive airway pressure) may be used to help your baby breathe. These devices provide oxygen through either nasal prongs, a face mask, or a special tube going through the nose or mouth into the baby's lungs.

Apnea

Apnea means not breathing. Because of its immature system, the premature baby sometimes forgets to breathe. This occurs in approximately one-third of babies born prior to the thirty-second week. Preemies who are at risk are monitored with special devices that sound an alarm to the nurses if the baby stops breathing. A nurse stimulates the baby by tickling its feet, its legs, or its tummy. This type of stimulation is often enough to start the baby breathing once again. Being present during one of these episodes may be frightening, but you should be confident that your baby is receiving the special care it needs. Your physician or nurse will tell you what to do should this happen when you go home.

Excessive Mucus

Excessive mucus accumulation is common among premature babies. If a baby is born prior to thirty-two or thirty-four weeks, it does not have an adequate cough reflex to remove the extra saliva that normally accumulates in the mouth. Eventually these secretions may enter the lungs, resulting in breathing difficulties and/or lung infections.

In certain instances, it may be necessary for a nurse to remove these secretions by suctioning with a soft, thin tube passed though your baby's mouth into the throat. It may be disturbing for you to see your baby uncomfortable for a few moments, but the benefits of this procedure outweigh the consequences of not removing the secretions.

Heart and Circulation

Birth produces many changes in a baby's circulatory system. In the womb, your baby's heart pumped blood throughout its body, including the placenta, in order to provide it with necessary oxygen. Because your lungs were breathing for your baby, blood bypassed the baby's lungs by a special valve called the ductus arteriosus.

Normally, this valve closes within twenty-four hours after birth, when the baby begins to breathe on its own. In the preemie, however, it may take longer for this valve to close, which may result in blood circulation problems. Failure of this valve to close is very common in babies with respiratory distress syndrome.

Heart Murmurs

If the ductus arteriosus is open and the blood flow becomes turbulent, the baby may have what is called a "heart murmur." A murmur is like the sound you hear when there is an obstruction in a quietly flowing stream. They are very common in the preemie and are often caused by this open duct. The duct usually closes as the baby matures; however, in some instances treatment may involve giving oxygen or medications or even performing surgery.

Jaundice

Jaundice is a yellowish discoloration of the skin and eyes caused by an accumulation of bilirubin in the bloodstream. Bilirubin is the normal end product when old red blood cells break down. In the mature system, the liver is responsible for removing this pigment, but in the newborn, the liver has difficulty ridding the body of all the bilirubin in the usual manner. If your baby has excess bilirubin in its system, its skin will appear yellowish.

The bilirubin level is determined by taking blood samples from a baby's heel. The treatment for a high bilirubin level is light therapy for a few days, either from direct sunlight or from special lights that help the body metabolize bilirubin. Your baby will be completely undressed, and its eyes will be protected from the bright lights. Be prepared for loose green stools. If the bilirubin level is very high, a blood transfusion may be necessary.

Anemia

Anemia is a deficiency of hemoglobin, the pigment in red blood cells responsible for carrying oxygen throughout the body. The preemie often has fewer red blood cells than normal. If your baby is anemic, you may find that it is paler than usual. A blood test confirms anemia.

Anemia is treated with a transfusion of red blood cells that have been specially screened for viruses and other potential disease-causing organisms. Your baby's blood type will have been determined at birth, and so immediate transfusion will be possible. Since most preemies already have an intravenous drip going, it simply means that the nurse or technician will have to add the bag of blood to the tubing—this involves no discomfort to the baby. Some very small babies may need more than one transfusion. You may find that following a blood transfusion your baby becomes more alert and energetic, in addition to having a better appetite and better color.

Some preemies are discharged from the hospital with iron supplements to be given by the mother. These iron supplements may cause your baby to have constipation and dark stools. Speak with your neonatologist or pediatrician about what is recommended for constipation.

Digestive System

The digestive system in the preemie is also immature. You will notice when you feed your baby that you must do so very slowly, because its stomach is very small. This is why frequent small feedings are often preferred.

Because of their immature system, many preemies do not digest their food properly. This may cause them to have a distended abdomen. Spitting up or regurgitation is also common because of the immature swallowing reflex. Holding preemies in the upright position after feedings or elevating the head of the mattress and putting them on their stomach or left side in their crib will help prevent them from aspirating these secretions into the lungs.

It is normal for a newborn to lose a few pounds during the first few weeks of life. This weight loss may last longer in the preemie. The preemie is usually maintained on intravenous solutions for a while and then is gavage fed (see below).

Feeding Problems

Feeding difficulties are probably among the most disturbing problems for parents visiting their newborn in the nursery. It may be frustrating for you when your little one either stops sucking or falls asleep while feeding. Eating is very tiring for your baby, and often feeding is done when the baby awakens by itself (demand-feeding) so that it can get all the sleep it needs. Preemies, in general, are not "demand" feeders, however; they will not tell you that they are hungry. So, in the beginning, feedings are usually given on a standard schedule. Do not be surprised if your baby falls asleep after or during feedings or if it has difficulty breathing after feeding.

One father comments,

> I vividly remember feeding our daughter the first week of life when my wife was recovering from her cesarean. Sometimes I would go to my daughter's bassinet, change her and pick her up, and she would still be asleep. My daughter had so little energy that the only way I could keep her awake during feeding time was undressing her and tickling her feet. Giving her one ounce of milk was a major task.

If preemies are born prior to thirty-two weeks of gestation, their sucking reflex will not be adequately developed. They will therefore be given gavage feedings, formula feedings given through a tube passing through their nose or mouth into their stomach. This tube may be left in place continuously or taken out and replaced intermittently. Because preemies do not yet have a gag reflex, they do not find this tube uncomfortable. Tube-fed babies are usually given pacifiers or nipple tops to suck on while being fed, so that they learn to associate sucking with feeding. An intravenous solution may also be inserted through a vein in their scalp to provide extra fluids and as a means of giving them any necessary medications.

Coordination of sucking and swallowing begins slowly to occur after the thirty-second week, but you may find that your little one continues to struggle until its thirty-fourth week. Some babies tolerate less food than others. If you are told that your baby is not tolerating its feedings, it means that the staff wants to reduce your baby's intake.

Necrotizing Enterocolitis

This is an inflammation or swelling in a section of the baby's bowel. It is not uncommon among premature babies and may cause the baby's abdomen to become swollen. It is most common in infants weighing less than 4½ pounds (2,000 g). The baby may have symptoms such as a distended, shiny abdomen, vomiting, and blood in its stool, sometimes accompanied by diarrhea. Successful treatment for this condition involves antibiotics and maintenance of adequate nutrition through intravenous therapy. Since this is an infection, care will be taken to ensure careful hand washing to prevent it from spreading to other babies in the nursery.

BREAST-FEEDING THE PREEMIE

Before your baby is born, you will probably have decided on a preferred feeding method. Babies tolerate breast milk more easily than formula, and breast milk contains special antibodies that help fight infections. The special bond and emotional fulfillment provided by breast-feeding make it a very desirable feeding method. However, as the mother of a preemie, you will find that the breast-feeding experience will have its share of both joys and frustrations. If your baby's premature birth came as a surprise or if your baby is in the premature nursery, breast-feeding may not be the most practical feeding method.

Breast-feeding a preemie is possible, but in most instances it requires attention and patience from you, the staff, and your family. In general, breast-feeding may be initiated in babies born after thirty-two or thirty-four weeks and weighing at least 3 lbs. 6 oz (1,500 g). A baby uses more of its own energy when breast-feeding, and therefore in smaller babies this method of feeding may need to be postponed.

When to begin breast-feeding is up to the individual mother and should be discussed with a nurse or physician. It depends upon your baby's health, your health, your baby's age, and the nursery structure—in other words, is there a quiet and relaxing room in which to initiate nursing? You will want to start breast-feeding as early as possible in your baby's life. Feeding sessions should initially be limited to ten or fifteen minutes at a time on each breast; the amount of time should be increased daily. If you are well, it is a good idea to offer the breast as much as possible during the day, even if it is just for a few minutes on each side. Some nurseries encourage nursing, while others believe that it is more important for the baby to rest.

Maintaining the milk supply is always a challenge for the mother of a preemie. The less your baby sucks, the less milk you will produce. Pumping will be necessary about every two to three hours to keep your milk flowing. Pumping is rarely enjoyable, but do not become discouraged if you are not producing a lot of milk. This is normal without the emotional fulfillment that you would get from holding your baby. To give yourself a sense a purpose, try pumping either near your baby or with a picture of the baby in front of you. Inquire if the nursery will allow you to store your milk in the refrigerator rather than discarding what may be beneficial to your baby.

There are many pumping methods—the manual method is the most popular and probably the least painful. Careful hand and breast washing cannot be overemphasized. Prior to nursing, you should massage your breasts starting at the top, and press firmly on your chest wall while moving your fingers in a circular motion. Do this all over the breast.

To manually express milk, place your thumb and forefinger in the shape of a "C" beyond the edge of the areola (about one inch from the nipple base). Press inward toward your ribs and then squeeze together, using pressure from the full length of your finger.

Some mothers choose mechanical pumping devices, which usually come with instructions. The milk is usually pumped for three to five minutes or until the flow diminishes. Electrical pumps may be less tiresome, but for some women they may be more painful. Pressure-cycled pumps may be more comfortable for some women. You can rent these devices from specialty shops, hospitals, or your local La Leche League.

Although there are some reasons why breast-feeding the preemie is not always successful even for the most determined mother, the main reason is the inevitable separation that occurs following the birth of a premature baby. As mentioned, preemies are often drowsy and breast-feeding is tiring for them; you may find yourself constantly trying to awaken your little one. Those of you who have had a cesarean may find it difficult getting into a comfortable position. Babies on oxygen therapy cannot be breast-fed, and women who have any type of infection are not advised to breast-feed the premature baby.

Tips on Breast-Feeding a Premature Baby

1. A preemie nipple may be used prior to feeding to initiate the sucking process.

2. Try keeping the drowsy baby awake by unwrapping some clothes, rubbing the soles of the feet, or stroking the throat under the chin.

3. Nurse the baby before it becomes too hungry. The hungrier they are, the less patience they have for nursing.

4. Express some milk before initiating nursing so that the baby can smell the milk.

5. Apply warm compresses to the breast prior to feeding to stimulate milk flow.

6. Preemies are often more comfortable nursing lying down in bed rather than in a chair. Take note of what your baby likes best.

7. Keep a chart of how long your baby nurses on each breast and how much formula it takes with each feeding. This gives you an idea of your progress. The less formula your baby takes, the more it is getting from the breast.

8. Give the bottle only after nursing. If that does not work because the baby is very hungry, offer a little bit before nursing to calm the stomach, and then nurse.

9. Take a rubber nipple and cut off the pointy part to make a nipple shield. Now you've got the best of two worlds (your baby's preferred rubber and your own nipple).

10. Wean the baby from the bottle as soon as possible.

11. Join a support group or speak to other mothers of preemies to share ideas and concerns.

YOUR FEELINGS

Life with a premature baby is filled with feelings of fear and uncertainty and a sense of urgency. You learn to take each minute and each day one at a time. You often wonder if your baby will survive. A baby's health status can change for better or worse within moments, as you will quickly learn. One woman comments,

> After the early birth of my baby at seven months, I really felt as if I had failed. I had a history of one stillbirth and felt like I was failing again. I really felt incapable of taking care of my daughter. Breast-feeding her in the nursery made me feel like I was contributing to her care. I believed it was so important to let her know that we loved her. I stayed in the nursery all day and my husband stayed there all night. At times the staff took it personally, thinking that we didn't have confidence in their care—but I really felt that it was the right thing to do. We felt she really needed us.

It is normal for you to go through a series of grief reactions following the birth of your preemie. You might think about the perfect baby you imagined during your pregnancy or you might have feelings of guilt for having borne a child one step short of "perfect."

Some parents may feel depressed and even erroneously and prematurely begin planning for a life of rearing a child with a disability.

It is very important to express your feelings and concerns with the staff and with your family and friends. Most parents have mixed feelings about having a preemie. Some couples are brought closer during these difficult times, while others find the strain too great and their relationship shatters. In the latter situation, one partner is unable to give emotional support to the other because both are so shocked and hurt by the event.

Going home without your baby is likely to be painful, and it is even more disconcerting if you live far from the hospital. When our baby was in the premature nursery, we rented an apartment nearby so that we could visit frequently and could be there quickly in the event of an emergency. Visiting your baby is very important. Even at such an early age, the baby needs to know that someone cares and that there are special people there on a regular basis. Your voice will probably elicit a reaction from your baby because it has been hearing it since early in your pregnancy.

Your role as the parent of a preemie rests in conveying a sense of hope to your newborn, who despite its problems manages to pick up all the signals—good and bad—that you send out.

Stimulating Your Baby

○ Keep in mind that infants like geometric shapes and respond best to black-and-white images or contrasting colors.

○ Place all objects approximately eight inches away.

○ Stimulate for short periods—they tire easily.

○ Talk to your baby.

○ If visiting is a problem, prepare a tape of your voice for the nurses to play.

○ Use eye contact.

○ Close its fist around a soft toy.

○ If possible, change the position of the crib periodically for a different view.

○ Remember that the best stimulation for your baby is seeing your face.

FAMILY AND FRIENDS

The birth of your premature baby will be considered a crisis in all your personal relationships. It is normal for it to affect everything you do. It is particularly difficult when the birth of a preemie comes without warning and you have no chance to prepare yourself.

Your partner will play a major role in your ability to cope. If you stand together and support each other rather than becoming angry and resentful, it will be much easier.

I remember how supportive my husband was during this time. We had a two-year history of infertility problems, and so the birth of our first daughter was wonderful beyond words. We put all our energy into helping her survive those first critical weeks of life. My husband was my "Rock of Gibraltar." In addition to being my replacement in the nursery, he made an effort to be with my daughter as much as possible, and especially made it a point to be there at feeding time to give her bottles. We learn a lot about our family during these difficult times. We learn whom we can depend upon when we need them, who is there and who is not.

Siblings are sometimes allowed to visit the premature nursery. Fostering this early interaction is very important. Depending upon the age of your other children, it may be difficult for them to understand the crisis situation. Explain as much as you think they will understand without overwhelming them. If you are at home and want to visit your newborn, find alternative care for your other children, especially if they have any type of infection—even if it is just a common cold. Preemies are very vulnerable to any type of infection because their immune system is underdeveloped.

Grandparents of preemies often need a great deal of support and explanation. Nurseries with restricted hours may make them feel left out. This is particularly difficult if it is a first grandchild. In many instances the grandparents feel even more excluded if there are other children at home and they are not directly involved in their care either.

Researchers have noted that grandparents feel triple grief, as they grieve for their new grandchild, for the infant's parents, and

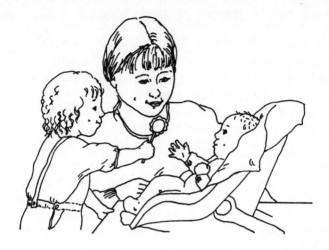

for themselves. Although they have this triple stress, in general they are more understanding of the necessary restrictions on visiting, and deal more easily with these limitations than do the parents. This may be traced to their own child-rearing period in the 1950s and 1960s, when even healthy full-term babies were shown in the nursery behind glass windows. In some instances, such as in the case of single parents, grandparents may play a large role in offering support to the mother.

OUTCOME

Today, the prognosis for babies born prematurely is much better than it was years ago. It depends upon many factors, including any complications during their first days of life and the type of care they receive. Many cities have high-risk units specializing in the care of these vulnerable infants. The presence of highly trained professionals helps to give parents confidence that everything is being done to ensure the best possible outcome for their baby.

In general, the smaller the baby, the less chance there is for survival and the more obstacles it will confront. Babies weighing more than 3 lbs. 6 oz (1,500 g), with good respiratory patterns and good muscle tone, have an almost normal chance of survival.

BABY'S HOMECOMING

Bringing your baby home will probably be one of the most exciting yet apprehensive days in your life, second only to learning
you were pregnant. Knowing that your child has survived the
trauma and the potential dangers of early birth gives you an enormous amount of strength. You may be overwhelmed that your
baby is finally coming home. You may also be scared and unsure
about your parenting abilities. It is important that you ask all the
pertinent questions about caring for your baby and also get a telephone number for the hospital, your pediatrician, or a local community agency, which you can use to ask any questions as they
arise. Some women find it helpful to join local support groups to
share the experiences of parenting a premature baby. This also
decreases the sense of isolation parents feel during the first difficult months of their baby's life.

Coming home with your baby will no doubt have a dramatic
effect on your family life. Having had your baby in the premature nursery will seem like a dream. Running back and forth to
the hospital and attending to your household probably gave you
little time to think about anything else. Once at home, you will
realize that the experience of having a premature baby is physically and emotionally exhausting. It is normal for the frustrations and anxieties to come to the forefront. Speak openly with
your spouse and request the same from him. Venting frustrations
rather than exhibiting generalized anxiety will prove healthier
in the long run.

Equipment needed at home for the premature infant is similar to that for term babies, with a few exceptions. Items such as
disposable preemie diapers are available in certain areas. The
manufacturer of Pampers™ has a premature-size diaper. Call
Procter & Gamble toll-free at 1-800-543-4932 to see where you
can purchase them in your area. Speak with other mothers of
preemies about where to buy preemie clothes or check out the
Internet for product information and suggestions. Most car seats
are designed for larger infants; however, you can adapt a standard
car seat by placing rolled towels on either side of your baby's head
for additional support. Look for companies specializing in your
baby's needs. Children's Medical Ventures, for example, has
designed the Wee Fit ™ car insert specifically for preemies. Other

companies sell car beds that lie flat, allowing a premature baby with respiratory problems to breathe more easily. Be aware of air bag warnings and recalled products. And by all means, resist the temptation to hold your baby in your arms.

The first few days at home are the most difficult. You may find that the care you give your child is more tiring than you expected. If this is the case, perhaps a community agency or a visiting nurse can give you a hand. It takes a while for you and your baby to get used to each other. You will learn all the normal sounds that your baby makes during the night, and your baby will begin to adjust to its new home. One woman says,

> I was both terrified and delighted to take my baby home from the hospital after she had been there for four weeks. I kept thinking about the day that I saw her stop breathing in the nursery because she had mucus in her throat. I was well prepared should it happen at home, but I was quite overprotective for the first little while. We protected her from all dangers, including an abundance of visitors. We were very strict as to who could visit, and those who visited had to be very careful and wash their hands before coming near the baby. In the end, all the precautions paid off because now, at the age of six, she is a happy and bright little girl making both her parents very proud.

DEATH AND DYING

The possibility of your baby's death may have been in your mind from the very beginning. This is a realistic and a normal concern, since about half of all infant deaths that occur during the first month occur among premature babies. About half the deaths in preemies occur during their first day of life, so if you have already passed the first day, your baby's chances of survival are that much greater.

My son

He had a perfect body:
> everything a man would need,
> right down to his balls which seemed so big.
He had two.

Sure, he was small, but he was feisty—
    the nurses said he was feisty.
    He was fighting for every breath.
By evening he looked like a dark rose:
    Cyanotic, they said.
    I was beginning to forget what he looked like
    without all the tubes and wires
    running out from his body.
His breaths are shallow now,
    except for the machine breaths;
    the machine breaths are his best breaths.
Why isn't he fighting any more?
    The doctor says he needs to save his energy.
    For what? What happens next?
I know it's dark out now: Three A.M.
    It's still daytime in here,
    except it's quieter.
    The nurses seem less interested now.
I think it's quiet, but it's not.
    I hear heartbeats,
    and breathing.
    Machines are breathing;
    their hearts are beating.
Would it be better this way?
    Should he cash in now after seventeen hours
    or will he cash in at the wheel of a BMW
    at seventeen years?
Cash in? What has he invested?
    What have I invested?
    I know what his mother has invested.
    Will she ever invest again?
Would she even recognize him now?
    How quickly her emotions run,
    From intense pain,
    To immense joy,
    To fear, and back to pain.
Down the hall the babies are lined up
    in front of the windows for all to see;

> They pull the blind
> on the hallway windows here.
>   Bert Bunnell

Many parents of dying children feel the need to be by the child's side right until the end, while others have difficulty coping with the emotional impact, finding it all too intense. If your child dies and you feel like hugging and cuddling it, you should be encouraged to do so. The tubes and apparatus are usually removed after death, so they should not interfere. Ask the staff for special tokens of your baby, such as name tags, armbands, or a lock of hair. If you haven't given your child a name, you may want to. Most nursery staff will give you an opportunity to spend time with your baby. No matter how short your baby's life has been, a bond has been formed between you, a special bond that will live with you forever.

Sometimes siblings have a difficult time adapting to the loss. They may need extra love and attention at this time. Here's a cartoon from *Frogs Have a Baby: A Very Small Baby,* by Jerri Oehler, R.N., at Duke University Medical Center.

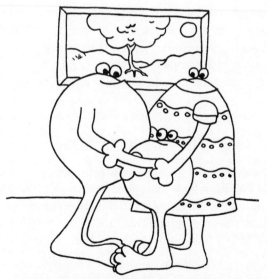

We will be here with you. It will take awhile to stop hurting and feel better. We love you and will take care of you. It's important to know that there will always be someone to love you and take care of you.

FUTURE PREGNANCIES

Before you leave the hospital or on your first visit to the pediatrician, you may still have many unanswered questions about why your baby was born prematurely and if it can happen again. It is important for you to voice your concerns. The risk of having another preemie is about 50 percent for those with severe kidney disease, severe hypertension, or proven uterine abnormalities.

Most authorities agree that you should wait at least three months before becoming pregnant again, especially if the premature birth resulted in the death of the baby. This is the minimum amount of time needed to accept your loss and to come to grips with your situation. For older women, this waiting may be difficult, as they are fighting the time element dictated by the remaining years of fertility.

Some women choose to change physicians and/or hospitals, while others prefer to stay with the old and familiar. This is up to the individual, and you should discuss your concerns with both your partner and your physician.

Depending upon your situation, you may be categorized as high-risk in your subsequent pregnancy. Make sure you understand what this means and whether you are in the same or a similar risk category as before. Although high-risk pregnancies are not something most women want to repeat, there is no doubt that the second time around is much easier, as you will know more what to expect.

HELPFUL RESOURCES

Preemiewear, specializes in clothing for preemies or low-birthweight babies. To order a free catalog call (800) 992-8469.

Tiny Bundles, offers unique handmade preemie clothing, diapers, and pacifiers. To order a free brochure call (619) 451-9907, or write to 11438 Ballybunion Square, San Diego, CA 92128.

Chapter 13

———————— O ————————

Preventing Birth Defects

According to the March of Dimes Birth Defects Foundation, a birth defect is "an abnormality of structure, function, or body chemistry, whether genetically determined or the result of environmental interference before birth. It may be present at or before birth, or appear later in life." In 1985, more than 250,000 infants in the United States had birth defects resulting in physical or mental damage. Today, birth defects affect more than 150,000 babies annually, remaining the leading cause of infant death. In other words, one out of every five infant deaths is due to a birth defect. Approximately 3 percent of infants have malformations and 1 percent have multiple malformations. Some are more serious than others, but no defect is easily accepted by parents. Many months of imagining the "perfect baby" are suddenly shattered.

A study by Beckman and Brent concluded that 15 to 25 percent of birth defects are caused by genetic diseases or chromosomal abnormalities. Approximately 8 to 10 percent are caused by environmental factors such as maternal infections, diseases, and exposure to chemicals or drugs. The remaining 65 percent of birth defects are caused by unknown reasons or may be due to many factors (multifactorial).

A teratogen is an agent that may cause a birth defect. Some examples of teratogens include chemicals, drugs, infections, and diseases. The most vulnerable period for the fetus is during the first two months, when the basic organ systems of the body are being formed. After this, the principal occupation of the fetus is growth. Thus, the chances of the fetus being affected are greater if your exposure was during a critical period of its development, such as the first trimester.

The actual effect of the teratogen will depend upon a number of variables, including the fetus's vulnerability, when you are exposed, the nature of the teratogen, the dosage, and your general health.

Some Possible Teratogens

Accutane
Alcohol
Caffeine
Tobacco
Drugs
    anticonvulsants
    coumadin
    DES
    illegal drugs
    methotrexate
    oral hypogylcemics
    retinoids
    thalidomide
Infections
    cytomegalovirus
    rubella
    toxoplasmosis
Venereal diseases
    AIDS
    chlamydia
    gonorrhea
    herpes
    syphilis
Environmental and occupational hazards
    DDT
    lead pollution
    poor nutrition
    video display terminals (VDTs)
    X-rays

To discuss each teratogen in detail is beyond the scope of this book. Therefore, I have chosen to discuss the most common teratogens and those that affect us all—if not every day, then at

some time during our pregnancy. A detailed discussion of infections and venereal diseases can be found in chapter 5. The effects
of poor nutrition are discussed in chapter 6.

DRUGS AND PREGNANCY

In adults, the kidney and liver are responsible for facilitating the
breakdown of medications and their excretion from the body. In
the fetus, the kidney and liver are immature, and therefore the
mother's liver and kidney take on this responsibility. Drugs that
are considered mild, such as aspirin, may be potentially harmful
to the unborn child. In general, the most hazardous time to take
any drugs—prescribed, over-the-counter, or street drugs—is during the first three months. This is why you should begin prenatal
care early.

Probably two of the most publicized teratogenic drugs are
thalidomide and DES. Thalidomide is now used only for Behcet's
Disease and as potential cancer treatment. It is a known teratogen and its use during pregnancy has been associated with multiple deformities. DES, a drug given to many women between 1941
and 1971 to prevent miscarriage, has resulted in certain female-
related cancers in the offspring of women treated with this drug.
Its use has been discontinued.

The best policy is not to take any drugs, prescription or non-
prescription, during pregnancy unless you and your physician
agree that it is absolutely necessary and that the benefits of the
drug outweigh the risks.

Illegal drugs

Drugs are labeled "illegal" when they are highly dangerous unless
taken under medical supervision. Some examples of illegal or
"street" drugs include crack and cocaine, heroin, morphine, and
amphetamines. Taken during the later part of pregnancy, these
drugs will cause withdrawal symptoms in the baby.

Crack and cocaine are the most dangerous drugs to take during pregnancy. Cocaine is a highly addictive drug whose usage has
increased dramatically in the United States in the past decade.
Approximately one in ten women use cocaine; this number may

be higher in urban centers. The federal government estimates that anywhere from 100,000 to 375,000 cases of cocaine-addicted newborns are reported yearly. The maternal use of cocaine has been linked with an increased risk for impaired fetal growth, spontaneous abortion, preterm labor, and abruptio placenta. Infants born of an addicted mother are inconsolable, and any effort to comfort them increases their agitation. Sometimes sedation is required in the early moments of life. Developmental damage to the baby is severe. The mother should seek help following the birth and should link up with a special treatment program.

The National Institute on Drug Abuse has established a hotline to provide treatment referral and general information about cocaine. Pass this number on: 1-800-662-HELP.

ALCOHOL AND PREGNANCY

Alcohol is potentially dangerous to the unborn child, as it is capable of crossing the placenta and entering the fetal bloodstream; therefore, concentrations found in the fetus are at least as high as those in the mother. Thus, if the pregnant woman is an alcoholic, there is a greater risk of having a complicated pregnancy.

No "safe" amount of alcohol consumption during pregnancy has been established, so it is recommended that pregnant women simply avoid it. What researchers do know is that six drinks per day (3 oz each) constitute a major risk. The timing of alcohol ingestion is also very important. It appears that the most dangerous time to consume large amounts of alcohol is in the first and last trimesters. During the first trimester there is rapid fetal cell growth, and in the last trimester there is rapid brain growth.

When a person ingests more alcohol than the liver can process, the excess is released into the bloodstream, where it circulates until the body is able to detoxify it. Alcohol present in a pregnant woman's body is distributed in the fetal liver, pancreas, kidney, thymus, heart, and brain. Alcohol has the ability to affect fetal growth during pregnancy because it interferes with carbohydrate, fat, and protein metabolism, thus retarding cell growth.

The most serious adverse effect of excessive alcohol consumption during pregnancy is fetal alcohol syndrome (FAS). Babies with this syndrome are born with a low birth weight and unusual facial features, such as small eyes, a flat nose, and uncommon eye folds. Many also have various types of heart, skeletal, and genital problems. Death in the early newborn period is not uncommon, and those who survive have borderline to moderate mental retardation.

Fetal alcohol effect (FAE) is the name given to alcohol-induced developmental impairment that entails anything less than FAS. It is often more difficult to diagnose and for this reason may be more widespread in the general population. Studies have shown that although children with FAE may appear normal, their learning ability is impaired. In a mild case of FAE, for example, the child may show a repeated failure to understand his or her multiplication tables, may also have difficulty mastering certain social skills, or may have poor judgment. These children may also have difficulty learning from their mistakes.

The subject of FAS was addressed in the 1989 book *The Broken Cord* by Michael Dorris. The story it tells about the dramatic effects of alcohol abuse on a pregnancy is both revealing and inspiring. The author presents the story of his adoption of a Sioux Indian who turns out to be afflicted by FAS. The trials, anger, and joy of raising such a child are all addressed.

If you drink wine or liquor every day and are contemplating pregnancy, it is a good idea to consider quitting or to seek help before jeopardizing the health of a future child.

CAFFEINE AND PREGNANCY

To date, the exact effects of caffeine on pregnancy are unclear. However, studies have shown that in very high quantities, caffeine may negatively affect pregnancy. This is because caffeine is absorbed by both mother and child. Caffeinated foods such as coffee, tea, cola, and chocolate should all be used in moderation during pregnancy. If you feel tired and need a boost, it is much better to get some rest. More than one cup of coffee a day is not recommended during pregnancy, especially if you prefer strong coffee.

Coffee activates your system and encourages stress hormones such as epinephrine and norepinephrine to be released, affecting blood flow and the amount of oxygen available to the fetus. Many women make the wise choice to use decaffeinated beverages and substitute herbal teas for regular teas. Heavy coffee consumption is also often associated with cigarette smoking, and the two together are sometimes used to substitute for the snacks between meals that are much needed by the pregnant woman.

TOBACCO AND PREGNANCY

In 1996, 13.6 percent of American women who gave birth were smokers. According to the Center for Disease Control, tobacco use has fallen steadily since 1989, when about 20 percent of pregnant women smoked. Nevertheless, smoking remains a problem. Smoking is hazardous during any stage of life, but is particularly hazardous for the pregnant woman. Studies have shown a strong correlation between moderate to heavy smoking (one pack per day) and low-birth-weight and premature babies. Growth retardation and low birth weight can indicate the beginning of other problems in the newborn. Some other problems that may be traced to smoking include premature rupture of the membranes, abruptio placenta, maternal hypertension, prematurity, and miscarriage. Some studies also indicate that children born to smokers are more likely to suffer infections of the respiratory tract, such as bronchitis and colds, and may be more susceptible to SIDS.

If you already have a high-risk pregnancy due to any of these problems and continue to smoke, you are exacerbating your situation. Recent studies have shown that not only is it harmful for smokers to smoke, but it may be detrimental for nonsmokers to be in the presence of smokers. This is an important consideration for the pregnant woman.

ENVIRONMENTAL HAZARDS

Little is known about how the fetus is affected by the external environment. Nuclear fallout, as experienced after the Chernobyl and Three Mile Island mishaps, clearly has an effect on the frequency of miscarriages and fetal abnormalities. During these kinds of environmental disasters, pregnant women and nursing mothers are advised to stay indoors.

Pregnant women are also advised to avoid routine chest and dental X-rays in order to minimize the chances of causing any harm to the fetus. Hospital X-ray departments often have posters on the walls advising pregnant women against having unnecessary X-rays. If you have any questions, ask about any treatment that is recommended for you.

Lead exposure has been linked to low birth weight and impaired speech, memory, learning, and intelligence. Although there has been a swing to unleaded fuel, it is recommended that pregnant women try to avoid rush hour and traffic jams to minimize any possible exposure.

Paint removed from buildings built prior to 1978 contains lead particles that may be very toxic. Those who are involved in making jewelry or stained glass where lead solder is used should avoid these hobbies, as they could raise a woman's blood lead level.

For most adults, however, our diet is our major source of lead. Food may be contaminated as a result of lead deposits from the atmosphere on crops. Vegetables grown in urban gardens near old painted structures may be another source. Studies indicate that coffee and alcohol consumption is associated with increased maternal lead levels. It is known that dietary supplements of calcium, iron, and folic acid can lower blood lead levels. However, these should only be taken under medical supervision.

OCCUPATIONAL HAZARDS

Certain work environments may also be hazardous to the unborn child. This is certainly true for hospital personnel, especially those who work in the operating room and are in close proximity to anesthetic gases. A man's sperm count may be reduced by these gases, and a fetus may be vulnerable to certain congenital abnormalities. Ventilation systems may help to minimize the risks, but the best way to avoid them if you either are trying to become pregnant or are already pregnant is to remove yourself from these workplace hazards. It is important to avoid benzene (a known cause of cancer), paint fumes, and other chemical fumes.

Another source of concern has been the use of video display or computer terminals (VDTs) by the pregnant woman. Some isolated studies have shown that VDT users may face a higher risk of birth defects and miscarriage. Long-term studies are still under way; however, a recent review does not support these findings.

VDTs produce small amounts of X-rays, but the glass screen tends to block virtually all of it. Remember, though, that radiation is emitted from the back and sides of the terminal; you may want to speak to co-workers about rearranging your desks. In general, most scientists agree that VDTs are safe, except those manufactured prior to the 1970s. The guidelines below have been provided by the Office Technology Education Project in Boston.

Tips on Minimizing Risks from VDTs

○ Limit hours at the VDT (less than twenty hours per week).

○ Turn off your computer when not in use.

○ Avoid sitting next to a laser printer.

○ Sit at least four feet from your terminal when you are not using it and you must keep it on.

○ Avoid using old equipment.

○ Take frequent breaks to avoid stress.

HELPFUL PUBLICATIONS

Cocaine Use During Pregnancy
VDT Facts
Drinking During Pregnancy
Single copies of these pamphlets are available from:
The March of Dimes Foundation
Community Services Department
1275 Mamaroneck Avenue
White Plains, NY 10605

While you are writing, remember to request their "Catalog of Public Health Education Materials" or call 1-800-MODIMES for more information.

Chapter 14

——————————— O ———————————

Genetic Risks

There are many possible causes of birth defects, and often the problems are due to hereditary factors, environmental hazards encountered during pregnancy, or a combination of both, or to untraceable errors in development. The following sections will discuss affected babies in terms of the genetic, environmental, and multifactorial causative factors. A short discussion of genetics will help to explain the discussions of the actual diseases that follow.

GENETICS AND PREGNANCY

A human being originates from the union of two gametes, the ovum and the sperm. These cells contain half the inherited characteristics (genes) of each parent. Genes are arranged on rodlike structures called chromosomes, which bear each person's genetic material. Chromosomes occur in pairs and are present in every cell of the body.

At conception, there is a union of twenty-three of your chromosomes and twenty-three of your partner's (or one of each pair), giving your baby a total of forty-six chromosomes in every normal cell. Twenty-two pairs of these chromosomes are called autosomes and are the same in males and females. The twenty-third pair, however, are called the sex-determining chromosomes. Females have two X chromosomes and males have one X and one Y. These sex chromosomes determine not only sex but also certain diseases that may affect either males or females.

Genes are the basis of heredity, and they may be thought of as the storehouse of information that determines how your baby develops. Your and your partner's genes, as they interact with environmental factors, form the picture of your child's characteristics, including his or her physical appearance, health status, and life span. It can be said that genes serve to join the past and the present to the future.

Who Is at Risk?

During one of your earliest prenatal visits, you will be asked whether there is any family history of genetic problems. Any physical or mental problems among family members should be mentioned, including miscarriage, stillbirth, and early infant death. If there is a history of an inherited problem you may be referred to a genetic specialist for further investigations.

We are all at risk for genetic problems, but certain couples are more at risk. They include:

○ Those with a genetic condition themselves

○ Women who have had a stillbirth or a live birth with a genetic condition

○ Those who have a family history of a genetic abnormality

○ Women who are suspected or known carriers of sex-linked disorders (e.g., hemophilia, muscular dystrophy)

○ Women who have phenylketonuria (PKU)

○ Couples who are blood-related

○ Women over the age of 35

○ Women who have had two or more miscarriages

It is amazing how much must go right in order to bring a healthy child into the world! What is surprising is that more errors do not occur during the reproductive process. Spontaneous losses, such as in the case of the blighted ovum discussed earlier, do occur.

Genetic disorders fall into three major categories: chromosome, single-gene, and multifactorial. Approximately 7.5 percent of all congenital malformations are due to single-gene defects; 6 percent are due to chromosomal problems; 28.5 percent are multifactorial; and nearly 60 percent are due to what experts call unknown factors.

CHROMOSOMAL DEFECTS

In general, chromosome problems are caused by errors in cell division. The type of abnormality may be the result of either too much genetic material or too little. Unlike single-gene defects, which may reoccur with subsequent pregnancies, chromosomal defects most often are caused by the amount of genetic material transmitted and so affect only a specific pregnancy. Some chromosomal defects may be hereditary; therefore, this possibility needs to be explored with each individual family. Approximately 1 infant in every 150 to 200 is born with a chromosomal abnormality. Downs syndrome and Turners syndrome are two examples; the former is the most common chromosomal disorder in live-born infants.

Downs Syndrome

Downs syndrome (mongolism, or Trisomy 21) is a congenital condition characterized by varying degrees of mental retardation and multiple physical defects. The incidence of Downs syndrome, as indicated below, depends upon maternal age. It is most often caused by the presence of an extra number 21 chromosome.

Mother's Age	Risk of Downs syndrome
25	1 in 1,250
30	1 in 952
35	1 in 378
40	1 in 106

If you are over the age of thirty-five, your physician will suggest either an amniocentesis or chorionic villi sampling to verify the number of fetal chromosomes (see chapter 7).

Many pregnancies in which the fetus is affected with Downs syndrome result in miscarriage, but those babies who survive vary in their capabilities. Half of these children will have heart problems, and some will have problems involving the bowel, blood, or other body systems. The most outstanding physical features include upward-slanted eyes, small ears, and a protruding tongue because of an undersized mouth. Mental retardation is common and may range from mild to severe. An encouraging and stimulating environment helps these children develop to their fullest potential.

Turners Syndrome

This is a less common chromosome abnormality, occurring in about 1 in 2,500 to 3,000 females, where one X chromosome is abnormal or absent. The condition affects only females, and there may be few symptoms in the newborn period. In some cases, however, the baby may have puffy hands and feet, a webbed neck, and cardiac problems. Later in childhood, the girl may have short stature, late breast development, and lack of menstrual periods because of small ovaries. These girls need to take hormonal supplements throughout puberty. Unfortunately, they are almost always sterile. Otherwise, they can lead a normal, full life.

SINGLE-GENE DEFECTS

Single-gene defects occur when a change or a mutation involves one or both of a single pair of genes. Autosomal dominant means that the abnormal gene will dominate over the "normal" one. A dominant condition is one in which only one member of the pair of genes needs to be altered in order for the condition to be expressed. The condition may be passed from generation to generation, with the risk of inheriting the gene being 50 percent (see diagram). For example, if one parent has high cholesterol with a predisposition to heart disease, there is a 50 percent chance that the offspring will have heart disease. Some rare dominant disorders are listed below. Detailed discussions are beyond the scope of this book.

○ Achrondroplasia (dwarfism)

○ High blood-cholesterol levels

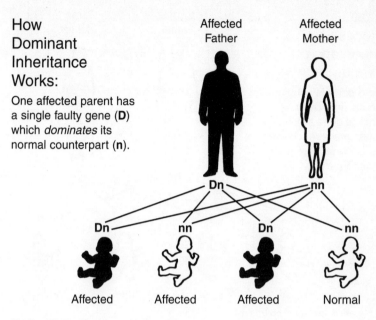

How
Dominant
Inheritance
Works:

One affected parent has
a single faulty gene (**D**)
which *dominates* its
normal counterpart (**n**).

Affected
Father

Affected
Mother

Dn   nn

Dn   nn   Dn   nn

Affected   Affected   Affected   Normal

Each child's chances of inheriting either the **D** or the **n** from the
affected parent ar 50%.

How Dominant Inheritance Works

(Courtesy of March of Dimes Birth Defect Foundation)

○ Huntington's chorea (progressive neurological deterioration)

○ Osteogenesis imperfecta (very brittle bones)

○ Polydactyly (extra fingers or toes)

○ von Willebrand disease (poor blood clotting)

A recessive gene problem is one that manifests itself only
when both members of the gene pair are abnormal. Usually both
parents have one copy of the abnormal gene and yet are healthy
themselves. A child who receives an autosomal recessive gene from
both parents shows its trait. For example, having blue eyes is a
recessive trait. Recessive genes are rare, and so the chance of mar-
rying a carrier of the same genetic disease is unlikely if you marry
outside of your family. All of us are carriers for some recessive conditions. Our children have problems only if our partner is also a

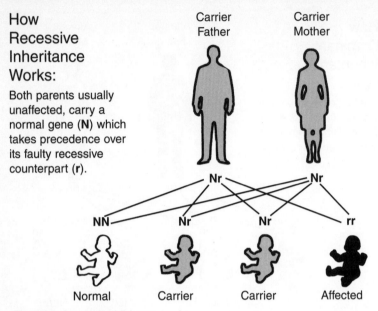

How Recessive Inheritance Works:

Both parents usually unaffected, carry a normal gene (**N**) which takes precedence over its faulty recessive counterpart (**r**).

Carrier Father   Carrier Mother

Nr   Nr

NN   Nr   Nr   rr

Normal   Carrier   Carrier   Affected

The odds for each child are:
1. a 25% risk of inheriting a "double dose" of **r** genes which may cause a serious birth defect
2. a 25% chance of inheriting two **N**s, thus being unaffected
3. a 50% chance of being a carrier as both parents are

How Recessive Inheritance Works

(Courtesy of March of Dimes Birth Defect Foundation)

carrier; as a result they inherit two copies of the harmful gene. When both parents are carriers, the risk with each pregnancy is 25 percent (see diagram). Some examples of recessive disorders are

o Beta-thalassemia (blood disorder)

o Cystic fibrosis (affecting secretions in lung and pancreas)

o Galactosemia (inability to metabolize milk)

o Phenylketonuria (PKU)

o Tay-Sachs disease (fatal neurological disease)

The most common recessive disorders are discussed below.

Sickle-Cell Anemia

Sickle-cell anemia is an inherited hemoglobin disorder that primarily affects people of West African origin. Children who receive the gene from both parents have predominantly sickle-cell hemoglobin, which causes their red blood cells to become deformed because they are deprived of oxygen. As a result, they may suffer from anemia, which may range from mild to severe. They may have "sickle-cell attacks," which are caused by the passage of these deformed red blood cells through the capillaries (the smallest blood vessels in the body). There is no cure, and death may occur during an acute crisis due to a severe infection or health problem. Sickle-cell anemia may be detected prenatally. Those with a family history of this disorder should seek genetic counseling prior to considering pregnancy.

Cystic Fibrosis

This is an inherited recessive disorder affecting about one in two thousand newborn Caucasian children. It is a metabolic disorder that affects the mucus glands of the body and results in thick secretions. The bodily systems that are affected include the lungs and the pancreas. The disease is often recognized early in life. The infant may have a chronic cough, foul-smelling stools, difficulties metabolizing sugar, and heat intolerance. Chronic lung infections are common due to the thick lung secretions, which serve as a nourishing medium for bacterial growth.

Cystic fibrosis is transmitted to a child when both parents carry the recessive gene but do not have the disease. There is a 50 percent chance that the child will just carry the gene and a 25 percent chance that the child will be unaffected.

There is no cure for cystic fibrosis, and it is usually managed at home. The standard treatment is to deal with the symptoms as they arise with the help of antibiotics, to liquefy the characteristic thick secretions, and to provide aggressive physical therapy to keep the lungs free of secretions. Detecting cystic fibrosis prenatally can be done through amniocentesis, chorionic villi sampling, and analysis of genetic material. Today, testing is reserved for known carrier couples who have a one-in-four risk of having a child with cystic fibrosis, or those with a close family history. After birth, cystic fibrosis is diagnosed with a sweat test, which measures the amount of salt in the sweat.

Phenylketonuria (PKU)

This is a rare recessive condition affecting one in twelve thousand births in the United States. It is discussed here primarily because every newborn is tested for this condition. It is most frequent in those of Northern European origin. PKU is characterized by the child's inability to process or metabolize the amino acid phenylalanine. One consequence of this is the excessive production of phenylketones, which are excreted in the urine. The disruption of phenylalanine metabolism can prevent the child's brain from developing properly and can lead to severe mental deficiencies, behavior disturbances, and sometimes seizures.

Infants born with PKU appear normal for the first few months. Those who are not treated begin to lose interest in their surroundings by the age of three to five months. By the time they are one year old, they show progressive mental retardation accompanied by physical symptoms such as dry skin, foul-smelling urine, skin odor, and very fair hair. Treatment, which must be initiated within the first few weeks of life, is with a special diet giving only the necessary amount of phenylalanine. With this diet, which needs to be followed at least until adolescence, a child can progress in a normal or near-normal manner.

Today, newborns are routinely tested for PKU within two days after birth in the hospital. A small amount of blood is taken from the baby's heel to see if there are abnormal amounts of phenylalanine. If the baby is premature or is born at home, arrangements are often made for the same screening. If you have PKU and were treated as a child, your own child may be at risk during pregnancy. If a woman with PKU is not maintained on a strict diet before and during pregnancy, the high levels of phenylalanine may cause a miscarriage or increase the risk of having a child with PKU symptoms, even if the child is only a carrier of the gene.

Tay-Sachs Disease

This disease is an autosomal recessive disorder resulting in progressive deterioration of the neurological system. The symptoms include loss of interest in the child's surroundings, loss of muscle tone, and poor head control, all of which may appear between three and six months of age. When the child is eighteen months old, he or she may become deaf and blind and have uncoordinated muscle movements. These children usually die of a respiratory infection by the time they are three to five years old. The disorder is most common among those of Eastern European Jewish ancestry.

Tay-Sachs can be detected by a routine blood sample taken from a pregnant woman, but the test is not done unless specifically requested. When both of the parents are carriers, prenatal diagnosis is available by amniocentesis and/or chorionic villi sampling, and at that time the couple may decide on continuing or terminating the pregnancy if the fetus is affected. There is no cure for this tragic disease, and the treatment is merely to support the child and to treat the symptoms as they arise.

SEX-LINKED DISORDERS

Sex-linked or X-linked defects are traits usually carried on an X-chromosome. There are many X-linked disorders. The traits may be either dominant or recessive; the latter are more common. In X-linked recessive disorders, a woman may be a carrier of the disease or defect that is manifested only in her male children. If you are a carrier of an X-linked disorder, the risk for a male or female to inherit the abnormal gene is 50 percent. The females will be carriers, while the males will be affected (see figure on page 247). Some examples of X-linked recessive disorders are

○ Agammaglobulinemia (lack of immunity to certain infections)

○ Color blindness

○ Duchenne-type muscular dystrophy

○ Hemophilia (bleeder's disease)

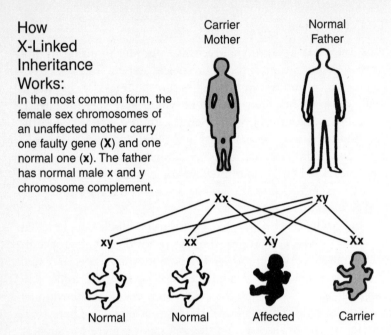

How X-Linked Inheritance Works:

In the most common form, the female sex chromosomes of an unaffected mother carry one faulty gene (**X**) and one normal one (**x**). The father has normal male x and y chromosome complement.

Carrier Mother — Xx

Normal Father — xy

xy — Normal

xx — Normal

Xy — Affected

Xx — Carrier

The odds for each *male* child are 50/50:
1. 50% risk of inheriting the faulty **X** and the disorder
2. 50% chance of inheriting normal x and y chromosomes
For each *female* child, the odds are:
1. 50% risk of inheriting one faulty **X,** to be a carrier like mother
2. 50% chance of inheriting no faulty gene

How X-Linked Inheritance Works

(Courtesy of March of Dimes Birth Defect Foundation)

MULTIFACTORIAL DISORDERS

Many inherited problems are caused by a complex interaction of genetic and environmental factors. These are called multifactorial disorders. The incidence of some of these disorders is low, as is the chance of them recurring in subsequent children. Some examples of multifactorial disorders are

○ Cleft lip/cleft palate

○ Club foot

○ Congenital hip dislocation

- Some congenital heart defects/diseases '

- Congenital scoliosis

- Some diabetes mellitus

- Hirschsprung disease (congenital large colon)

- Hydrocephalus (water on the brain)

- Mental retardation

- Spina bifida (open spine)

- Pyloric stenosis (narrowed/obstructed opening from stomach to small intestines)

- Some urinary-tract malformations

MUTATIONS

Certain environmental factors may cause a chemical change in the gene, resulting in mutations. Mutations occur spontaneously in the population. In the laboratory, mutations can be caused by certain types of radiation, such as X-rays. Nuclear tests and accidents, like Three Mile Island and the Chernobyl incident in the Soviet Union, are a source of concern for geneticists. The effects of these disasters may be felt in future generations.

X-rays are not recommended during pregnancy. Although the normal dose of a routine X-ray do not necessarily cause harm, the effect depends upon the amount and time of exposure, and no amount of exposure to X-rays can be considered safe. The usual dosage of X-rays is one to three rads. Some sources state that exposure to more than ten rads during the first three weeks of pregnancy can result in miscarriage or in a smaller-than-usual brain size. There is no statistical evidence of abnormalities occurring when the mother is exposed to less than ten rads, but it is always recommended that she shield her abdomen from radiation.

If you do not think you are pregnant and need to have an X-ray, you should schedule it during your menses or within ten days of it. A man should also refrain from planning conception for six to eight weeks following an X-ray of the lower abdomen or genitals.

GENETIC COUNSELING

Many couples seek genetic counseling long before they try to conceive a child. Women who are at or over the age of thirty-five are the most frequent candidates for genetic counseling. The counselor has special training in hereditary diseases and in birth defects in general, and he or she may be a physician or a health professional specially trained for the task.

The genetic counselor will need to know about the hereditary diseases in your family, the causes of death of family members, and any stillbirths or miscarriages in your family. It is important that you bring forward as much information as possible. Talk to your family members to gain a thorough picture of your family history. If you already have an affected child, he or she needs to be investigated. To help the counselor understand the potential risks you face, he or she may recommend various diagnostic tests, including blood and skin tests. If you are already pregnant, you may be advised to have certain prenatal diagnostic tests, such as amniocentesis and ultrasound, to detect fetal defects. If you are planning to use in vitro fertilization, a preimplantation genetic diagnosis (PGD) may be offered. During the IVF procedure, clinicians perform a biopsy on the embryo. At this stage, many genetic disorders can be detected, allowing the couple to decide which embryo to implant.

Your counselor will discuss with you what has been ascertained from all the information gathered. Your family history will be drawn in the form of a pedigree chart that illustrates your family tree and any diseases of its members. The risks, if any, to yourself and/or your offspring will be discussed with you in detail. This information should, with your counselor's help, assist you in making an informed reproductive decision. Couples face difficult issues when genetic disease or its real possibility is present. All these factors are considered during the counseling sessions.

YOUR EMOTIONS

Learning that your child is affected is probably one of the most painful and stigmatizing experiences in your life. As one mother of a hemophiliac said, "No matter how it is presented, the fact of serious chronic illness is always difficult to accept."

A single mother observed,

> At first, I was in total despair. It somehow seemed to me that I couldn't do anything right. First, I had failed as a wife and now as a parent. But in the long, dark night that followed the disclosure of the news, I had a real change of heart. As an only child, I had been very much protected and I realized this was not standing me in good stead in life. I now realize that I was at a real crossroads. I could have either continued being a weak person, now with a perfect excuse of a very sick child, or I could grow up that minute—take charge of a new baby and my own life—and do something about my son and get moving. I did grow up that night and it is a decision I never regretted.

Early in your pregnancy, you and your partner began to imagine what your child would be like. This image was carried throughout your pregnancy, up to the birth of your child. After learning of your child's disability, it is normal for you to feel inadequate and helpless. It is normal to fear the reaction of loved ones, including grandparents, who may have long awaited the birth of this child. These feelings may be magnified if you have had infertility problems.

It is normal to feel your faith shaken. You may ask yourself questions like "Why did this happen to me?" "What kind of world is it in which such pain can be inflicted on people?" "Is there any meaning to our suffering?" One woman who cared for a daughter with hydrocephalus until she died at six years of age states,

> She was our only child and we did everything for her, including feeding, dressing, and bathing, because of her physical and mental handicap. She could not walk or sit or even talk to us. We accepted that she would never be normal and that we would do everything in our power to make her life as comfortable as possible. That was the decision we made.

In Rayna Rapp's article in Ms., "The Ethics of Choice," she writes about learning through amniocentesis that her fetus had

Downs syndrome. She discusses decisions women must make when they find they are carrying a handicapped fetus:

> Making the medical arrangements, going back for counseling, the pretests, and finally, the abortion, was the most difficult period in my adult life. I was then 21 weeks pregnant, and had been proudly carrying my expanding belly. Telling everyone—friends, family, students, colleagues, neighbors—seemed an endless nightmare. But it also allowed us to rely on their love and support during this terrible time. . . . Our community was invaluable, reminding us that our lives were rich and filled with love despite the loss.

Whatever decision you make regarding your baby-to-be, these will be difficult times for you. If you decide to have an abortion, it is normal to take a while to get over your loss. You may continue to wonder if you made the right decision or you may feel comfortable knowing that you were correct. If you decide to care for the child yourself, you should be prepared for the unavoidable strain the handicap will place on you and your family. You should also be prepared for society's reaction to your handicapped child. It is common for society to set you apart and make you feel different. It will be your own creative efforts that will make the difference in combating the loneliness often felt by handicapped people and their families.

HELPFUL PUBLICATIONS

Congenital Heart Defects
Down Syndrome
Single copies of these pamphlets are available from:
The March of Dimes Foundation
Community Services Department
1275 Mamaroneck Avenue
White Plains, NY 10605

Genetic Disorders
American College of Obstetricians and Gynecologists
ACOG Distribution Center
P.O. Box 4500
Kearneysville, WV 25430-4500

Chapter 15

—— O ——

Issues, Ethics, and Decision Making

Medical knowledge in all fields is growing at an enormous rate. Students who enter medical school today are told that much of what they learn will be obsolete by the time they graduate. Physicians and consumers alike must keep abreast of all these rapid developments.

Women are bearing children today who years ago would have had to settle for life without children. Babies are being born who just a decade ago would not have survived. This chapter will briefly discuss some of the progress made in our time and offer glimpses of developments. Many of the techniques discussed are used only in certain parts of the United States. Most medical advances are put into practice in large and innovative metropolitan clinics and hospitals before they become common practice in obstetrical science generally. There is a good chance that by the time you read this book there will be many further developments and pertinent issues on the medical frontier.

SINGLE MOTHERS

Some women unexpectedly become single mothers because of the death of a spouse from disease, accident, or war. Others become single mothers because of a divorce. However, there is another group who call themselves "single mothers by choice."

For the most part, these are women who have decided to have or adopt a child knowing that they will be the sole parent. They have varying backgrounds, according to the support group

SMC (Single Mothers by Choice), and many are career women in their thirties and forties. Some have decided after establishing their careers that they want to become mothers. Others have always had a strong mothering instinct and, as their biological clock ticks on, they choose not to wait for marriage before starting their family. Many of these women want "to have it all"—a career, the single life, and a child.

Women may become mothers in numerous ways. Some may become pregnant accidentally, some intentionally, others choose artificial insemination, and yet others may choose to adopt.

There has been a definite increase in single motherhood over the years: 18 percent between 1980 and 1985. In 1990, 170,000 single women over thirty gave birth.

TEENAGE PREGNANCY

In 1996, an estimated one million teenagers became pregnant, resulting in 494,272 babies. One-third of those pregnancies ended in abortion. According to Child Trends Inc. (1990), teen mothers tend to come from disadvantaged backgrounds, so part of their difficulty as parents stems from the fact that they are more likely to be poor even before becoming parents. As few as three in ten teen mothers are married and live with their husbands. Another half live with relatives, and an additional one in twenty live with both their husband and other relatives.

There has been an increased infant and maternal mortality associated with adolescent pregnancy. Therefore, pregnant teenagers need both physical and mental prenatal care. Ideally, it would be best to prevent teenage pregnancies. This may be done through educators, employers, and community policy makers. Their combined efforts may help to control recurrent teenage pregnancy. When pregnant for the first time, a teen is often seen as a high risk for a subsequent pregnancy and should be counseled so that she does not become pregnant again.

Groups such as the National Organization of Adolescent Pregnancy and Parenting, Inc., in Bethesda, Maryland, serve as networks dedicated to preventing adolescent pregnancy and the many problems related to it.

SEX SELECTION

Modern medical science raises many ethical questions, but perhaps no other arouses as much interest and controversy as determining the sex of your child. For centuries people have used superstition to predict the sex of an unborn child or have offered suggestions on how to choose the baby's sex.

There are various reasons why couples want to choose the sex of their child. First, there is increased awareness of over two hundred known sex-linked genetic disorders whose appearance is linked to whether the child is a boy or a girl. In families known to be at risk for an X-linked condition, sex selection may be an alternative. Others feel that they only want to have a child if it could be the sex that they prefer.

Sex determination has always stirred a great deal of controversy. Dr. Roberta Steinbacher, a social psychologist, conducted a study at Cleveland State University and found that if a proven technique were available, about 25 percent of couples would take advantage of it. In the same study, 91 percent of the women and 94 percent of the men said they would prefer that their firstborn be a boy. Others say that sex selection would decrease population growth because couples often have more children than they want while trying for their sex of choice.

For those who have had infertility problems, the sex of the child may be irrelevant—a baby is what they want. But others believe that as long as the technology is available, why not use it?

More than six hundred children have been born in the United States using sex selection. There are many modes of sex selection. Some are practiced by couples at home, while others are performed in the laboratory. Most techniques are based on the premise that the male determines the sex of the child.

Home-Based Sex Determination

The male chromosome is the Y and the female is the X. To have a boy, there must be an X and a Y chromosome. To have a girl, two X chromosomes are united. The male-producing or Y sperm have been identified as being smaller and often faster, under ideal conditions, than the female-producing or X sperm. The

X sperm are characterized as being more resistant to various types of stress.

Based on these facts, Dr. Landrum Shettles, a pioneer in sex selection and coauthor of the book *How to Choose the Sex of Your Baby*, says that there are a number of facts a couple can keep in mind when trying to determine the sex of their child. First, because the male-producing sperm are faster, they will probably reach and fertilize the egg first when intercourse occurs at or near ovulation, when secretions are more alkaline and favorable for sperm penetration. The larger, female-producing sperm will most probably fertilize an egg when intercourse occurs a day or so prior to ovulation, when the secretions are more acidic and more likely to eliminate the Y sperm. Therefore, the timing of intercourse is thought to be one way to influence sex selection.

There are other less proven methods, such as douching with a mild acid douche of two tablespoons of white vinegar to one quart of warm water prior to intercourse to increase the chances of having a girl, and a douche of two tablespoons of baking soda in a quart of warm water to increase the chances of a boy. If you use these techniques, you are still taking your chances with probability.

Laboratory-Based Techniques

There are also laboratory methods of sex determination that utilize the difference between the X and Y sperm. They are based on the separation of male- and female-producing sperm in the laboratory to produce the sex of choice. Typically, the male's semen is washed in a tissue medium and then run through two glass columns containing viscous layers of human serum albumen (protein medium). When the sperm have descended to the bottom, they are removed and separated from the liquids around them. The sperm of the chosen sex are then concentrated and injected into the woman's cervix shortly after ovulation. Producing females in the laboratory is more difficult than producing males. The procedure costs from $200 to $300 and is offered in many clinics throughout the United States.

The procedure is not 100-percent effective. One woman who had five girls went to a clinic desperate to have a boy. To her surprise, she ended up nine months later with another girl.

Another similar procedure uses a centrifuge to separate X- and Y-bearing sperm. Since the female chromosome is heavier, it sinks to the bottom. The Y or male chromosome floats to the top. Doctors then perform artificial insemination using the isolated sperm, according to the parents' preference.

The majority of couples who seek these interventions want a male child. Although these techniques can be used for nonmedical reasons, there may be a place for these procedures in certain X-linked conditions in order to prevent the chance of a male fetus.

FETAL SURGERY

For some, fetal surgery is a possible alternative to abortion or to the birth of a handicapped child. In the laboratory, fetal surgery on animals has been used for more than three decades. In fact, the removal by fetal surgery of certain body parts of animal fetuses has been the basis of many research projects on fetal growth. The answers provided by this research have given investigators explanations for problems occurring in pregnant women, while at the same time suggesting ways to treat many congenital abnormalities.

Fetal surgery in humans began in the 1960s with intrauterine red blood cell transfusions for those with Rh problems. Prior to the advent of this procedure, the fetus would have died of such complications as anemia and swelling (edema). Since ultrasound was introduced in the 1970s, it has been used to diagnose certain problems that may benefit from surgery after twenty-four weeks of pregnancy. By the early 1980s, fetal surgery was being used to treat fetal blockages by the insertion of a catheter or tube through the mother's uterus to facilitate adequate drainage of excess fluids. Today, most types of fetal surgery involve the use of a catheter passed into the mother's abdomen.

In 1981, Dr. Michael Harrison, at the University of California at San Francisco, did the first "open fetal surgery," where the woman's uterus was opened and the fetus was exposed, to treat a severe fetal blockage in the urinary tract (hydronephrosis).

In general, most fetal anomalies are left to be treated, either medically or surgically, until after birth. In some cases, however, surgical intervention may be recommended in utero. These situations include cases where the fetus's problem is getting worse with time and may eventually lead to its death. Thus far there have been three major problem areas in which fetal surgery has been attempted: congenital hydronephrosis, congenital diaphragmatic hernia, and sacrococcygeal teratoma.

Congenital Hydronephrosis

Congenital hydronephrosis, or urinary-tract obstruction, prevents kidneys from developing normally and causes a blockage in the urine flow. It usually develops early in pregnancy and affects the ureters and urethra. In severe cases, the mother usually has less amniotic fluid because the fetus is not excreting the normal amount of urine. The fetus's lungs are also poorly developed because they are dependent upon fluid for their growth and development. Those with severe forms of the disease detected early in pregnancy would be good candidates for surgery, but only after a very thorough medical assessment.

During an ultrasound, a small catheter is placed into the fetal bladder to temporarily drain the urine into the amniotic fluid to remove any obstruction. The tube is left in until after birth, when surgery is done to correct the blockage. The fetal mortality rate from this procedure is about 4 percent, and the survival rate following birth is close to 50 percent. The mortality rate from the disease itself is much higher if left untreated.

Congenital Diaphragmatic Hernia

In this congenital abnormality, the fetus does not have a complete diaphragm, and therefore the stomach, small intestines, and other organs slip into the fetus's chest, crowding the lungs and interfering with proper development. At birth, the baby's lungs are so small that it is unable to breathe. The incidence of diaphragmatic hernia is about 1 of every 2,200 births. About 50 percent of these fetuses die, often in the delivery room. Until now, the usual treatment has been to wait for birth, attach the newborn to a respirator, and then operate on the hernia as soon as possible.

With the help of ultrasound, diaphragmatic hernias may be detected and treated early with fetal surgery. However, only about 10 percent of fetuses are suitable for this type of surgery.

This surgery is still being performed at various centers, although some babies who don't have this surgery in utero also can do quite well.

In 1990, Dr. Michael Harrison performed his first successful diaphragmatic repair. The mother was twenty-four weeks pregnant. The surgeons made a small incision in the mother's womb, lifted aside the fetus's left arm, opened the baby's chest, and pushed the abdominal organs into their proper place. The fetus's diaphragm was then closed with a patch of Gore-Tex (the waterproof material used in parkas). The operation took less than one hour, and seven weeks later baby Blake was born. For the first three weeks of his life he was on a respirator; at the time of this writing he was at home and doing very well. In March 1991, Dr. Harrison performed similar surgery on a little girl who is also doing well.

Sacrococcygeal Teratoma

Sacrococcygeal teratoma is the most common type of congenital tumor that may affect the newborn. This occurs in about one out of every forty thousand births; 80 percent of babies with this condition are females.

The decision whether to perform fetal surgery is not an easy one for the physician or for the couple. All the variables must be considered, including the severity of the defect and the chances of a successful result.

THE FETUS AS PATIENT

Now that practitioners have found ways to see and treat the unborn child, they are faced with complex decisions. Today, both mother and child are considered patients during pregnancy. Medical advances may help fetuses survive who, under "normal" circumstances, would not have had the gift of life.

Ethical, legal, and economic questions will continue to be raised as long as medical technology advances at such an unrelenting pace. Questions are being posed about the rights of both the mother and the fetus. A procedure will be advocated if it is beneficial to mother as well as to child. If either the mother or the baby is put in danger as a result of the procedure, it will probably not be performed.

Ethical questions arise when the mother waives her right to have fetal surgery. Is it her right to decide? Who makes the decision? Can we make analogies with the choice to have a cesarean or an abortion? In a 1987 article in *Current Problems in Obstetrics, Gynecology, and Fertility*, Dr. Sherman Elias and Professor George Annas state that society should honor a mother's refusal of intervention, since we assume that the mother has the fetus's best interest in mind. In the journal *Nursing Clinics of North America* (1989), author J. G. Twomey argues that court resolutions of such situations should be reserved for situations in which the mother and father disagree or the mother's competence or judgment is in question. The author goes on to say that adequate prenatal care helps reduce the very problems that may force the mother to contemplate fetal surgery.

There are also certain dilemmas from an economic standpoint. The cost of surgical intervention is high, but so is the medical care required for a child with severe defects. Caring for the chronically disabled is very costly, especially if it is necessary to keep these children institutionalized.

Although surgical intervention can help many, a certain risk is always present and must be weighed against the benefits. Careful assessment of the fetus by a skilled team is essential before the decision is made to recommend fetal surgery. The fact that a procedure can be done does not always mean it should be done.

Although professionals may believe intervention to be necessary, you, the parents, have the right to decide what you think is best for your unborn child, based on all the information that you have gathered. The best decision is an educated one. Whatever you decide for your unborn child, you can be thankful that today you have the option to choose sophisticated interventions, a choice parents of previous generations never had!

MAKING DECISIONS

The first choice for a mother-to-be is the decision to become pregnant. For some, especially those following career paths, that may be the most difficult decision they have to make. Making decisions involves much more than sitting down one evening and saying, "Okay, now I'm going to decide." For most people it involves weeks or months of ongoing thought about the choice. It involves interactions and conversations with family, friends, and professionals. Your choice will depend upon your ethical beliefs and principles as well as your financial status at the time.

After the decision to become pregnant is made, a woman needs to choose a physician, a hospital, whether or not to have tests, whether to breast-feed, and so on. If she is at risk, she will continuously be making decisions concerning both her own and her baby's health. If she is over the age of thirty-five, she will decide whether she wants to have an amniocentesis. If the results of the amniocentesis indicate problems, she will have to decide whether to have an abortion. This decision is probably the most difficult of all to make, since no one wants to terminate a potential life. Raising a child with disabilities, on the other hand, may be more than some women can contemplate.

The best decisions are educated and informed ones. When you must make a choice, it is important that you gather all the information you need. Sit down with paper and pencil and write out the pros and cons. Consider all the factors. Make a list of all the alternatives you have in the given situation. It is important to solicit the ideas and opinions of family, friends, and experts. Gathering and thinking over other people's viewpoints will help you come to your own, personal decision. Then you will know that you have made a truly caring and wise choice for yourself—and for your unborn child!

Appendix A

─────────── O ───────────

The Reproductive System

This section will describe the female and male reproductive systems and fertilization. A clear understanding of these processes and the associated terminology will be of great help in communicating with your caregivers and will give you a greater sense of control in your decision making.

The Female Reproductive System

The External Anatomy

When looking at the female reproductive system externally, one sees the vulva, a term that includes all the visible sexual parts. There are two sets of folds that protect the vagina: the labia majora (outer folds) and the labia minora (inner folds). When the folds are spread apart, one sees the clitoris, urethra, vaginal opening, and two pairs of lubricating glands.

Labia Majora These outer skin folds contain sebaceous glands that produce sweat and oil around the hair follicles that usually begin appearing in puberty. They also serve as a protective "door" to prevent infection and disease from entering the vagina and other internal organs. For some women, the color of this skin is darker than the inner folds, the labia minora.

Labia Minora These are exposed when the labia majora are pulled back. They have no pubic hair and fold directly over the vagina. They are very sensitive to touch. During sexual arousal, the veins of the labia minora become darker and constrict and grip the penis. This is perhaps nature's way of keeping the male's semen inside without spilling.

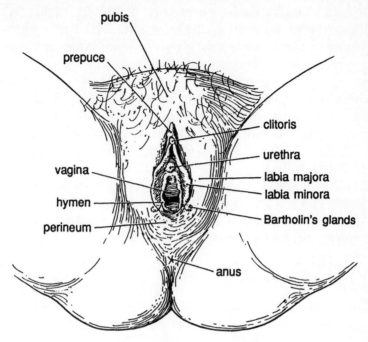

External Female Reproductive Anatomy

The labia minora also secrete a white lubricant called smegma, which should be washed away daily. The size of both labia vary; they seem to become larger and more stretched out with childbirth.

The clitoris lies at the upper portion of the genitals where both skin folds meet. It is the most sensitive spot in the entire genital area and is highly erotic. The clitoris is comparable to the male penis in terms of its ability to enlarge with sexual excite-ment. Its size and shape vary, and it may expand from ¾ inch to 1½ inches during sexual excitement.

Urethra This is the urinary opening or the tube that carries urine from the bladder out of the body. The tube is much shorter in women (about 1½ inches) than in men, and this is why women are more prone to urinary tract infections. Because the urethra is so close to the vagina, it is common for it to become irritated from prolonged or vigorous intercourse. Some women may feel discomfort during urination after intercourse. This may be alleviated by drinking one or two glasses of water before and after intercourse.

Lubricating Glands Two ducts, known as Skene's glands, are located on either side of the urethra. During sexual arousal these glands secrete a lubricating fluid. Another set of glands, called Bartholin's glands, are located under the labia majora. If there is any infection in the vulva it will easily be transmitted to the glands and cause an inflammation, which sometimes may swell to the size of a golf ball. If the gland becomes infected with bacteria, a cyst may develop that will have to be removed. This is a common spot for the gonorrhea germ to live.

The Internal Anatomy

The vagina is a muscular canal lined with mucus membranes extending from the vulva to the uterus, and it is sometimes referred to as the birth canal. It has many functions. It is the passage for the menstrual flow, it guides the penis and holds the semen near the cervix, and it serves as the birth canal.

The vagina is usually 4 to 5 inches in length and is very flexible. However, with age, sexual activity, and childbirth it tends to lose a lot of this flexibility. It secretes an odorless and watery discharge, sometimes clear and sometimes white. This lubricates the canal, keeps it clean, and helps maintain a slightly acid environment to prevent infections. Some women find that their vagina may become very dry or very wet. Drier times usually occur before puberty, during breast-feeding, after menstruation, and after menopause. Wetter times occur during ovulation, during pregnancy, and during sexual arousal.

In young girls, the entrance to the vagina is partially closed off by the hymen. Hymens come in different sizes and shapes, and for some women they stretch easily. The first time the hymen is stretched by sexual activity, little folds of hymen tissue will remain around the vaginal opening. Occasionally these are large and may have to be removed for comfort.

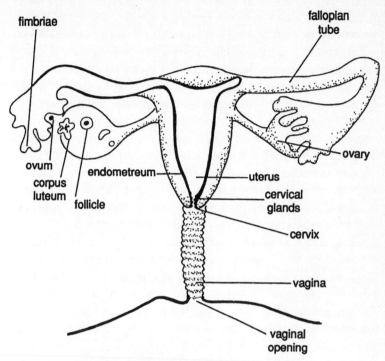

Internal Female Reproductive Anatomy

Pelvic Floor Muscles When you try to hold back your urine, you are contracting these muscles. They also serve to hold the pelvic organs in place and provide support for your other organs. If these muscles are weak you may have trouble reaching orgasm and controlling your urine flow (urinary incontinence), or have prolapsed pelvic organs (downward displacement of an organ from its usual position).

Anus This is the opening of the rectum, or large intestines, to the outside. The skin around the anus is very smooth, but sometimes external hemorrhoids (small varicose veins) develop after childbirth. It is important to keep the anus clean and to wipe from front to back to avoid getting fecal matter from the anus into the vagina.

Cervix This is a small rounded opening, about 1½ inches across, which separates the vagina from the uterus or womb. It is sensitive to pressure, though it has no nerve endings. Discomfort during intercourse is usually due to the penis hitting the cervix, which pushes against the uterus. The cervix changes position, color, and shape during puberty, the menstrual cycle, sexual excitement, and menopause. No tampon, finger, or penis can go through it, although it is capable of incredible expansion during labor and delivery.

The cervix plays a vital role in fertility. To prevent the entry of foreign matter, the cervix is blocked by a plug of mucus, and it is this plug that is vital in fertility. During ovulation, when the egg is released from the ovary into the fallopian tube, the mucus thins to allow sperm to swim past and reach the uterus. When the cervix is not healthy because of disease or injury, it is unable to control the quality and quantity of mucus, and this can affect fertility.

The uterus or womb is a flat, pear-shaped organ suspended in the pelvic cavity by strong bands of ligaments. When you are not pregnant, your uterus is about the size of a fist. It has very thick muscular walls, some of the most powerful ones in the body. The top of the uterus is called the fundus and is the most contractile portion of the uterus. The uterine muscles are strongly influenced by hormones each month. During menstruation, the uterine contractions are strong, and they are, of course, even stronger during childbirth.

Each month, the inner layer of the uterus is shed during menstruation, unless of course you are pregnant! If pregnancy does occur, then the embryo implants itself in the inner wall of the uterus (endometrium), which becomes a bed for the placenta.

The fallopian tubes, sometimes called oviducts or "egg tubes," extend outward and back from both sides of the upper end of the uterus. They are about four inches long and look like ram's horns facing backward. Inside, the tubes are lined with brushlike tips called cilia, which move the egg forward.

Each fallopian tube ends in the fimbria, fingerlike extensions composed of many separate petals, each one of a slightly different length and usually hanging down to the ovary.

The fimbria are vital in getting the egg from the ovary to the fallopian tube. There are various theories about how this occurs. One theory is that the egg drops onto one petal of the fimbria, which are covered with cilia cells that curl toward the inside of the tube. Another theory is that the fimbria sweep across the surface of the ovary and set up currents that wave the egg into the tube. In rare cases when the egg is not "caught" by the tube, it may become fertilized outside the tube, resulting in an abdominal pregnancy.

The fallopian tubes must be in optimum condition for fertilization to occur. They are extremely delicate, and this is why they are a major site of fertility problems.

The ovaries are two organs about the size and shape of unshelled almonds, located on either side of and somewhat below the uterus. This puts them about four or five inches below your waist. They are held in place by connective tissue and are protected by a surrounding mass of fat.

Ovaries have two functions: to produce germ cells (eggs) and to produce female sex hormones (estrogen, progesterone, and other hormones). When a baby girl is born, her ovaries contain about four hundred thousand immature ova; about four hundred of these will develop into mature eggs.

If for any reason a woman loses one ovary, the remaining ovary takes over the entire workload. This means it must produce one egg each month and double its hormone production. Ovarian disorders are also a common cause of infertility.

The Menstrual Cycle

Puberty is the time in a young girl's life when her reproductive organs mature. In general, puberty lasts about 1½ years, during which time the ovaries produce increasing amounts of the female sex hormone estrogen. This hormone is responsible for the female sex characteristics, such as breasts and body contours. It is also responsible for the uterus's development and helping the eggs to mature. Progesterone is also secreted and is responsible for the growth of pubic hair and the new intensity of erotic desire.

In combination, estrogen and progesterone cause the uterine lining to thicken and prepare for egg implantation—pregnancy. If pregnancy does not occur, the follicle dies, the progesterone level drops, and the uterine lining sheds. This shedding of the uterine lining is menstruation.

Menstruation usually begins between the ages of ten and sixteen. At this time the girl is physically capable of becoming pregnant. The usual amount of menstrual flow amounts to about four to six tablespoons of vaginal and cervical secretions, tissues,

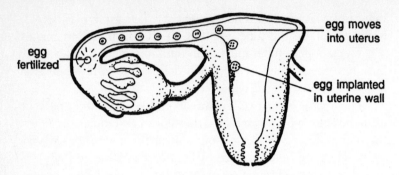

egg fertilized

egg moves into uterus

egg implanted in uterine wall

Fertilization and Implantation of the Egg

and blood. The length of time for each menses varies from a few days to a week. In the beginning, menstrual periods are very irregular while the body's hormones develop a pattern. After the first year or two, a pattern is seen; some may have a twenty-six-day cycle, while others may have a thirty-two-day cycle. Usually, the length of a woman's cycle remains the same, although this may be altered by stress, illness, a change in altitude, and so on.

The menstrual cycle has four phases: the bleeding phase—menstruation; the proliferative phase—the body prepares itself for pregnancy; the ovulation phase—the release of a ripe egg from the ovary; and the secretory phase—the secretion of progesterone and estrogen, which lasts for about fourteen days.

The growth and release of the egg and the growth and shedding of the endometrium are controlled by hormones. Understanding how hormones control fertility is important in understanding how fertility drugs help women become pregnant.

THE MALE REPRODUCTIVE SYSTEM

When a male baby is born, his penis is fully formed and his testicles have usually descended from the abdomen into the scrotal sac. All sexual organs are formed: the penis, testicles, scrotum, glands, and ducts.

The External Anatomy

The penis has two functions: to provide an outside port for urination, and to provide a means to get the sperm from the testes out

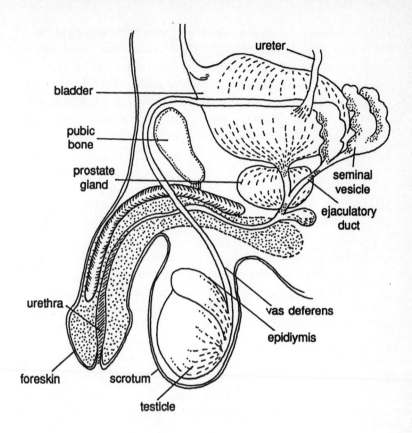

Male Reproductive Anatomy

of the penis into the vagina. The penis contains three cylinders of tissue surrounded by a tough fibrous covering. During sexual excitement, these tissues become engorged with blood, causing the penis to expand and become hard and erect. The most sensitive part of the penis is around the head, especially around the ridge that connects it to the shaft. During ejaculation, semen spurts out from the urethral opening at the tip of the penis.

The exact size of the penis is inherited. Large and small penises tend to run in families. Studies have shown that the size of the penis in no way affects sexual ability.

Some men are circumcised—the foreskin surrounding the penis is removed—while others are not. At one time this was done mainly for religious and/or cultural reasons, but over the years many have advocated the procedure for both hygienic and medical reasons. Some claim that the foreskin is a haven for bacteria, especially if proper hygiene is not carried out. If the circumcision is done at birth, it involves taking this fold of tissue (foreskin) over the tip of the penis and pulling, clamping, and cutting it. The incision is covered with an antiseptic gauze and usually heals within ten days. The need for circumcision remains a matter of controversy.

Scrotum and Testicles   There are scrotal sacs located on either side of the penis. Each protective sac contains one testicle, which is about two inches long and one inch in diameter. The primary functions of the testicles include production of testosterone (male hormone) and sperm. This is why it is important that they remain free from injury. During sports or strenuous activities it is recommended that men wear a jockstrap to provide the needed protection.

Perhaps nature's way of maximizing sperm production was to place the testes outside the body. To produce sperm, the testes prefer a cooler temperature. For some, fertility may increase in warmer weather, because when it is warm the muscles holding the testes relax and let the testicles drop away from the body. On the other hand, in colder climates the scrotal muscles contract and tend to bring the testes closer to the body.

The Internal Anatomy

Epididymis   This is a long hollow, coiled structure located just above the testicles, where sperm are matured and stored. The journey of the sperm through the epididymis takes three to twelve days, and by the end of the journey the sperm are completely matured. Mature sperm use the tail of the epididymis as a holding tank, and may remain here as long as one month. Not all of the sperm will live that long, however, and a man who ejaculates only once a month may have a high concentration of dead sperm and therefore a lower fertility rate. The epididymis is prone to infections, such as chlamydia, which can cause scarring and thus block sperm passage through the epididymis.

The spermatic cord is comprised of the vas deferens (see below) and a network of veins and arteries.

Vas Deferens These sperm ducts are two firm tubes that extend from the epididymis to the prostate. Mature sperm enter the vas and are gently squeezed along by the tube's pulsating walls. The sperm travel through these tubes and are stored at their upper ends until they mix with the seminal fluid—secretions from the seminal vesicles and prostate—just prior to ejaculation.

The combination of seminal fluid (98 percent) and sperm (2 percent) make up the semen, or ejaculate.

Seminal Vesicles These two glands store the sperm and contribute fluid to the ejaculate, secreting more than half of the ejaculate.

Prostate Gland This walnut-sized gland secretes an important chemical that causes the semen to liquefy. The secretions from the prostate comprise most of the seminal fluid or ejaculate and give the ejaculate its characteristic whitish color. This gland sometimes enlarges later in life, which may cause problems with urination.

Cowper's glands are two tiny glands located just below and in front of the prostate gland. They secrete a small amount of clear, sticky fluid that holds the sperm together and is sometimes visible prior to ejaculation. This fluid sometimes contains sperm; therefore, withdrawal from the vagina just prior to ejaculation is not a reliable means of birth control.

The urethra is the major channel of transport for both urine and sperm. It is a tube that runs from the bladder and down through the prostate gland where the ejaculatory duct empties into it, ending at the slit at the end of the penis. Both urine and seminal fluid travel through the urethra, but never at the same time. The body has an elaborate way of engaging the muscle that blocks urine flow during an erection.

Sperm Production (Spermatogenesis)

Sperm are not born—they are made. The process of spermatogenesis is coordinated by hormones produced by the testes and the hypothalamus, which is located above the pituitary gland. The hypothalamus initiates the process by releasing GnRH hormone to the pituitary, which secretes FSH and LH. These hormones encourage the release of testosterone.

The germ cells in the testes begin to mature and develop tails and are now capable of fertilizing an egg. For anywhere from ten to fourteen days, they are moved through the epididymis.

Ejaculation

Each man releases, on the average, sixty million or more sperm into the vagina with each ejaculation, each one carrying the necessary genetic information for the formation of a new person. Studies have shown that nearly 90 percent of these sperm are killed by vaginal secretions.

If intercourse occurs under optimal conditions, the sperm that survive can swim through the cervical canal within only twelve to twenty hours. Only a few hundred may reach the uterus, and many may go up the wrong fallopian tube. In the optimal conditions, the union of the sperm and the egg can occur within thirty-five minutes from the time of ejaculation. If ovulation is not happening, some sperm may continue to live in niches inside the fallopian tubes and wait for the egg, which may or may not come. Many specialists claim that sperm can live under these conditions for as long as seventy-two hours, possibly longer.

HOW PREGNANCY OCCURS

Each month during the woman's reproductive years, about ten to twenty ovarian follicles (small sacs, each containing an egg) begin maturing under the influence of hormones such as FSH (follicle-stimulating hormone), which is produced by the pituitary gland in the brain in the early phase of the monthly cycle. Usually only one follicle develops fully to release a mature ovum ready for fertilization; the others degenerate.

A few days before the follicle has reached its maximum size it secretes a large quantity of estrogen. This increased level of estrogen stimulates the cervix to produce a thinner mucus, which allows the sperm to enter the uterus. At the same time, this elevated estrogen stimulates the pituitary gland to release another hormone called LH (luteinizing hormone). The release of this hormone stimulates ovulation.

The follicle with the mature egg moves toward the surface of the ovary. At ovulation, the follicle disintegrates and the egg flows out. Some women may feel a twinge or cramp in the lower abdomen at this time.

The egg normally proceeds through one of the fallopian tubes, where fertilization occurs if there are sperm. If fertilization occurs, the fertilized egg travels down the fallopian tube for implantation in the uterus. The lining of the uterus must be both healthy and ready for implantation, and the body's hormones must be at an optimal balance for pregnancy to occur. In other words, the woman's body must be prepared for the pregnancy. There must also be both a healthy egg and a healthy sperm. If the egg is not fertilized, it is absorbed by the body and disappears, and menstruation begins.

Timing is very important for pregnancy to occur. It is important for the couple to have sex at the appropriate time in the menstrual cycle. Believe it or not, there are about five days each month when a fertile woman may become pregnant—the day she ovulates, about three days before, and one day after. In a twenty-eight-day menstrual cycle, ovulation usually occurs between day 14 and day 16. Regardless of the length of your cycle, if ovulation occurs, it will do so about fourteen days before menstruation begins. For example, if you get your menses every thirty-two days, you will ovulate between day 16 and day 20 of that cycle.

After the egg leaves the ovary, it lives for about twenty-four hours. Sperm live in your reproductive system for about three days after intercourse. If ovulation occurs within that period of time, you may become pregnant.

Once fertilization occurs, the egg, barely visible to the naked eye, floats freely in the uterus. It then begins to implant itself in the uterine wall to grow and develop. The fertilized egg is called an embryo at first and later on in pregnancy is called a fetus.

All eggs carry genetic information called chromosomes. These twenty-three pairs of chromosomes, combined with the twenty-three pairs from the sperm, create the potential for a new person. The chromosomes carried by the female are called the X chromosomes and those carried by the male are called the Y chromosomes. If the embryo is XX, it will be a female; if it is XY, it will be a male. This is why people claim that it is the male who determines the sex of the child.

Appendix B

———————— O ————————

Postnatal Exercise Program

The following exercises will help you get back on your feet as soon as possible after the birth of your baby. They are specifically aimed to help you

o Maintain good posture

o Prevent future back pain

o Strengthen abdominal, pelvic, and pectoral muscles

The exercises are to be done five times each, twice a day, for a six-week period after the birth of your baby.

Note: *Mothers who have had a cesarean can do all the exercises except Exercise 3, which should be started in six weeks to allow healing of the incision.*

Exercise 1: Pelvic Tilt

Lie on your back with knees bent, tighten your buttocks, and push your lower back into floor; hold two seconds. Relax.

Exercise 2: For Perineal Muscles

a) Lie on your back with your knees bent. Tilt your pelvis, squeeze your knees together, and tighten the muscles of the pelvic floor; hold for two seconds. Relax.

b) Practice stopping urination midstream by tightening your perineal muscles; hold for two seconds. Relax.

Exercise 3: For Abdominal Muscles

Lie on your back with your knees bent. Tilt the pelvis, tuck your chin in, and raise your head and shoulders as you

a) Stretch your hands toward your knees; hold for five seconds. Relax.

b) Stretch your hands to the outside of the right knee; hold for five seconds. Relax.

c) Stretch your hands to the outside of the left knee; hold for five seconds. Relax.

Exercise 4: Straight-Leg Raising

Lie on your back with one knee bent; lift the other leg up as slowly as high as you can; slowly bring it down.

Exercise 5: For Pectoral Muscles

Lie on your back. Press your hands together in front of your chest; hold for five seconds. Relax. Do this while lying down for breast engorgement.

Exercise 6: Pelvic Tilting in Standing Position

Stand with your back to a wall, feet one step away. Tighten your stomach, tighten your buttocks, and push your lower back into the wall; hold five seconds. Relax.

It is very important to do these exercises for the first six weeks after you have your baby. Your back is most vulnerable to the stresses placed on it at this time. Of course it would be beneficial to continue them for the rest of your life. The most important exercises are numbers 1, 2, and 3. Remember that good posture should be exercised at all times, whether you are sitting, standing, or sleeping.

(Modified with permission from Royal Victoria Hospital's Department of Physical Therapy, Montreal, Canada.)

Appendix C

Support Groups and Associations in the USA and Canada

INFERTILITY

Adoptive Families of America
2309 Como Avenue
St. Paul, MN 55108
(612) 645-9955
(800) 372-3300
www.adoptivefam.org

American Society for
Reproductive Medicine
(ASRM)
1209 Montgomery Highway
Birmingham, AL 35216-2809
(205) 978-5000
www.asrm.org

Center for Surrogate Parenting
8383 Wilshire Blvd. #750
Beverly Hills, CA 90211
(323) 655-1974
www.surroparenting.com

Creating Families, Inc.
1395 Bellaire Street
Denver, CO 80220
(303) 355-2107
www.creatfam.com

DES Action Canada
P.O. Box 233

Montreal, Quebec H3X 3T4
   CANADA
(514) 482-3204

DES Action USA National
   Office
1615 Broadway, Suite 510
Oakland, CA 94612
(510) 465-4011
(800) DES-9288
www.desaction.org

Endometriosis Association
8585 N 76th Place
Milwaukee, WI 53223
(414) 355-2200
(800) 992-3636
www.endometriosisassn.org

Ferre Institute Inc.
258 Genesee Street, Suite 302
Utica, NY 13502
(315) 724-4348
www.ferre.org

Fertility Research Foundation
875 Park Avenue
New York, NY 10021
(212) 744-5500

National Adoption Center
1500 Walnut Street
Philadelphia, PA 19102
(215) 735-9988
(800) TO-ADOPT
www.adopt.org

National Adoption Information
    Clearinghouse
330 L Street, SW
Washington, DC 20201
(703) 352-3488
(888) 251-0075
www.calib.com/naic

National Association of Surrogate
    Mothers, Inc.
P.O. Box 1927
Oceanside, CA 92051
(760) 430-1940
members.aol.com/nasmoms/home.
    html

National Cancer Institute
Cancer Information Services
Building 31, Room 10A19
Bethesda, MD 20892
(301) 496-4000
(800) 4-CANCER
www.nci.nih.gov

National Committee for Adoption
1930 17th Street, NW
Washington, DC 20009
(202) 328-1200
www.NCFA-usa.org

National Infertility Network
    Exchange
P.O. Box 204
East Meadow, NY 11554
(516) 794-5772

North American Council on
    Adoptable Children
970 Raymond Avenue, Suite 106
St. Paul, MN 55114
(651) 644-3036
members.aol.com/nacac

The Organization of Parents
    Through Surrogacy
P.O. Box 611
Gurnee, IL 60031
(847) 782-0224

RESOLVE
1310 Broadway
Somerville, MA 02144-1779
(617) 623-0744
www.resolve.org

HIGH-RISK PREGNANCY

American Diabetes Association
P.O. Box 25757
1660 Duke Street
Alexandria, VA 22314
(703) 549-1500
(800) DIABETES
www.diabetes.org

American Foundation for AIDS
    Research (AmFAR)

120 Wall Street
New York, NY 10005
(212) 806-1600
www.amfar.org

American Lupus Society
260 Maple Court,
    Suite 123
Torrance, CA 90505
(800) 331-1802

Center for Study of Multiple Birth
333 East Superior Street, Room
    464
Chicago, IL 60611
(312) 266-9093
www.multiplebirth.com

For Teen Moms Only
P.O. Box 962
Frankfort, IL 60423-0982
(815) 464-5465

International Twins Association,
    Inc.
6898 Channel Road, NE
Minneapolis, MN 55432
(612) 571-3022 / 571-8910

Mothers of Supertwins (MOST)
P.O. Box 951
Brentwood, NY 11717
(516) 859-1110
www.mostonline.org

National Diabetes Information
    Clearinghouse
P.O. Box NDIC
Bethesda, MD 20892
ndic@aerie.com

National Organization of Mothers
    of Twins Club, Inc.
P.O. Box 23188
Albuquerque, NM 87192-1188
(505) 275-0955
(800) 243-2276
www.nomotc.org

Parents of Multiple Births
    Association of Canada
P.O. Box 234
Gormley, Ontario L0H 1G0
    CANADA
(905) 888-0725
pomba.org

Triplet Connection
P.O. Box 99571
Stockton, CA 95209
(209) 474-0885
www.tripletconnection.org

Twin Services Inc.
P.O. Box 10066
Berkeley, CA 94709
(510) 524-0863
twinservices@juno.com

Twins Foundation
P.O. Box 9487
Providence, RI 02940-9487
(401) 274-8946
www.twinsfoundation.org

Twin to Twin Transfusion
    Syndrome Foundation
411 Longbeach Parkway
Bay Village, OH 44140
(440) 899-TTTS
www.ttsfoundation.org

Women and AIDS Resource
    Network (WARN)
30 Third Avenue, Suite 25
Brooklyn, NY 11217

NUTRITION

National Dairy Council
10255 West Higgins Road, Suite
    900

Rosemount, IL 60018-4233
(847) 803-2000

LOSS

Aiding a Mother Experiencing
  Neonatal Death (AMEND)
4324 Berrywick Terrace
St. Louis, MO 63128
(314) 487-7582

American Sudden Infant Death
  Syndrome Institute
6065 Roswell Road, Suite 876
Atlanta, GA 30328
(404) 843-1030
www.sids.org

Bittersweet Beginnings
(loss of multiple births)
5700 E Greenwood Place
Denver, CO 80222-5700
(303) 759-3979

Canadian Foundation for the
  Study of Infant Deaths
586 Eglinton Avenue E, Suite 308
Toronto, Ontario M4P 1P2
  CANADA
(416) 488-3260
www.sidscanada.org

Center for Loss in Multiple Birth
  (CLIMB)
P.O. Box 1064
Palmer, AK 99645
(907) 746-6123
www.climb-support.org

Compassionate Friends, Inc.
P.O. Box 3696
Oak Brook, IL 60522-3696
(630) 990-0010
compassionatefriends.com

Compassionate Friends National
  Center (Canada)

685 William Avenue
Winnipeg, Manitoba R3E 0Z2
  CANADA
(204) 787-4896

Helping Other Parents in Normal
  Grieving (HOPING)
Sparrow Hospital
P.O. Box 30480
1215 East Michigan Street
Lansing, MI 48909
(517) 483-3873
(810) 762-8801

Miscarriage, Infant Death,
  Stillbirth (MIDS, Inc.)
c/o Janet Tischler
16 Crescent Drive
Parsippany, NJ 07054
(201) 263-6730

National Council of Guilds
  for Infant Survival
(SIDS support)
P.O. Box 3586
Davenport, IA 52808
(319) 322-4870

National Sudden Infant Death
  Syndrome Resource Center
2070 Chain Bridge Road,
  Suite 450
Vienna, VA 22182
(703) 821-8955
www.circsol.com/sids

PEN Parents, Inc.
P.O. Box 8738
Reno, NV 89507-8738
(702) 826-7332
www.penparents.org

Pregnancy and Infant Loss Center
1421 East Wayzata Blvd., Suite 70
Wayzata, MN 55391
(612) 473-9372

RTS Bereavement Services
Gunderson/Lutheran Medical
    Center
1910 South Avenue
La Crosse, WI 54601
(608) 791-4747 ext. 4747
(800) 362-9567
berservs@gundluth.org

SHARE: Pregnancy and Infant
    Loss Support, Inc.
St. Joseph Health Center

300 First Capitol Drive
St. Charles, MO 63301
(314) 947-5616

Sudden Infant Death Syndrome
    Alliance
1314 Bedford Avenue, Suite 210
Baltimore, MD 21208
(410) 653-8226
(800) 221-SIDS
www.sidsalliance.org

Wintergreen Press
3630 Eileen Street
Maple Plain, MN 55359
(612) 476-1303
wpress@aol.com

CESAREAN BIRTH

Cesarean Support, Education and
    Concern (C/SEC, Inc.)
22 Forest Road
Framingham, MA 01701
(508) 877–8266

International Cesarean Awareness
    Network (ICAN)
1304 Kingsdale Avenue
Redondo Beach, CA 90278
(310) 542-6400
www.childbirth.org/ICAN

PREMATURE BIRTH

Federation for Children with
    Special Needs
95 Berkeley Street, Suite 104
Boston, MA 021116
(617) 482-2915
(800) 331-0688 (in MA)
www.fcsn.org

La Leche League International
1400 N Meacham Road
Schaumburg, IL 60173-4048
(847) 519-7730
(800) 665-4324 (in Canada)
www.lalecheleague.org

GENETICS

Alcoholics Anonymous World
    Services, Inc.
P.O. Box 459
Grand Central Station
New York, NY 10163

(212) 870-3400
www.alcoholics-anonymous.org

Alliance of Genetic Support
    Groups

4301 Connecticut Avenue, NW,
 Suite 404
Washington, DC 20008
(202) 966-5557 ext. 2304
(800) 336-GENE
www.geneticalliance.org

American Board of Medical
 Genetics
9650 Rockville Pike
Bethesda, MD 20814
(301) 571-1825
www.faseb.org/genetics

American Cleft Palate-
 Craniofacial Association
104 South Este Drive, Suite 204
Chapel Hill, NC 27514
(919) 933-9044
www.cleft.com

American Council for Drug
 Education
164 W 74th Street
New York, NY 10023
(800) 488-DRUG
www.acde.org

Association of Birth Defect
 Children
3201 East Crystal Lake Avenue
Orlando, FL 32806
www.birthdefects.org

Blind Childrens Center
4120 Marathon Street
Los Angeles, CA 90029-3584
(323) 664-2153
(800) 222-3567 (in CA)
(800) 222-3566 (in USA)
www. blindcntr.org

Canadian Cerebral Palsy
 Association

Wellington Street, Suite 612
Ottawa K1R 6K7 CANADA
(613) 235-2144
(800) 267-6572

Canadian Council of the Blind
P.O. Box 2310, Station D
Ottawa, Ontario K1A 8N5
 CANADA

Canadian Cystic Fibrosis
 Foundation
2221 Yonge Street, Suite 601
Toronto, Ontario M4S 2B4
 CANADA
(416) 485-9149
(800) 378-CCFF

Canadian Deaf-Blind and Rubella
 Association
P.O. Box 1625
Meaford, Ontario N0H 1R0
 CANADA
(519) 538-3431

Canadian Hard of Hearing
 Association
2435 Holly Lane, Suite 205
Ottawa, Ontario K1V 7P2
 CANADA
(613) 526-1584
(800) 263-8068
www.chha.ca/english.html

Canadian Hemophilia Society
100 King Street West
Hamilton, Ontario L8P 1A2
 CANADA
(416) 523-6414
www.hemophilia.on.ca

Canadian National Institute
 for the Blind
1931 Bayview Avenue

Toronto, Ontario M4G 3E8
    CANADA
(416) 480-7580
www.cnib.ca

Canadian Rehabilitation Council
    for the Disabled
Easter Seals/March of Dimes
    National Council
90 Eglinton Avenue E,
    Suite 511
Toronto, Ontario M4P 2Y3
    CANADA
(416) 932-8382
indie.ca/crcd

Cystic Fibrosis Foundation
National Center
6931 Arlington Road
Bethesda, MD 20814
(800) 344-4823
www.cff.org

Healthy Mothers, Healthy Babies
409 12th Street SW #309
Washington, DC 20024-2188
(202) 863-2458
(800) 322-2588

Juvenile Diabetes Foundation
    International
120 Wall Street
New York, NY 10005-4001
(212) 785-9500
(800) JDF-CURE
www.jdfcure.org

March of Dimes Birth Defects
    Foundation
1275 Mamaroneck Avenue
White Plains, NY 10605
(914) 428-7100
(800) 367-6630
www.modimes.org

Maternal PKU Collaborative
    Study
Division of Medical Genetics
Children's Hospital Los Angeles
4650 Sunset Blvd.
Los Angeles, CA 90027
(323) 669-2152

National Downs Syndrome
    Society Hotline
666 Broadway, 8th Floor
New York, NY 10012
(800) 221-4602

National Foundation for Jewish
    Genetic Diseases
250 Park Avenue, Suite 1000
New York, NY 10177
(212) 371-1030

National Genetics Foundation
555 West 57th Street
New York, NY 10019
(212) 586-5800

National Institute on Alcohol
    Abuse and Alcoholism
5600 Fisher Lane
Rockville, MD 20857
(301) 443-3860
www.niaaa.nih.gov

National Organization for Rare
    Disorders (NORD)
P.O. Box 8923
New Fairfield, CN 06812
(203) 746-6518
www.rarediseases.org

National Society of Genetic
    Counselors
233 Canterbury Drive
Wallingford, PA 19086-6617
(610) 872-7608
www.nsgc.org

Parents Helping Parents
3041 Olcott Street
Santa Clara, CA 95054-3222
(408) 727-5775
www.php.com

Parents of Downs Syndrome
Children
c/o Montgomery County
Association for Retarded
Citizens
11600 Nobel Street
Rockville, MD 20852
(301) 984-5792

Spina Bifida Association of
America
343 South Dearborn, Room 317
Chicago, IL 60604
(312) 663-1562

Turner's Syndrome Society
of Canada
814 Glencairn Avenue

Toronto, Ontario M6B 2A3
CANADA
(416) 781-2086
(800) 465-6744

Turner's Syndrome Society of
the United States
1313 Southeast 5th Street,
Suite 327
Minneapolis, MN 55414
(612) 379-3607
(800) 365-9944
www.turner-syndrome-us.org

United Cerebral Palsy
Associations
330 West 34th Street
New York, NY 10001
(212) 947-5770
(800) USA-5-UCP
www.ucpa.org

OTHERS

American Academy of Pediatrics
141 NW Point Blvd.
Grove Village, IL 60007
(847) 228-5005
www.aap.org

American College of Nurse-
Midwives
818 Connecticut Avenue, NW,
Suite 900
Washington, DC 20006
(202) 728-9860
www.birth.org

American College of Obstetricians
and Gynecologists
409 12th Street, SW
Washington, DC 20024-2188

(202) 638-5577
(800) 762-2264, ext. 199
www.acog.org

American Medical Association
515 North State Street
Chicago, IL 60610
(312) 464-5000
www.ama-assn.org

Association of the Care of
Children's Health
7910 Woodmont Avenue,
Suite 300
Bethesda, MD 20814
(301) 986-4553
(800) 808-ACCH
www.acch.org

Birthways
P.O. Box 12097
Berkeley, CA 94701-3097
(510) 869-2797

Canadian Diabetes Association
National Office
15 Toronto Street, Suite 800
Toronto, Ontario M5C 2E3
    CANADA
(416) 363-3373
(800) BANTING
www.diabetes.ca

Canadian Institute of Child Health
885 Meadowlands Drive,
    Suite 512
Ottawa, Ontario K2C 3N2
    CANADA
(613) 224-4144
www.cich.ca

Canadian Pediatric Society
100-2204 Walkley Road
Ottawa, Ontario K1G 4G8
    CANADA
(613) 526-3332
www.cps.ca

Centers for Disease Control
1600 Clifton Road
NE Building 1 South
Atlanta, GA 30333
www.cdc.gov

Consumer Information Center
Room G-142, (XC)
1800 F Street, NW
Washington, DC 20405
(888) 8-PUEBLO
(800) 688-9889 (Federal
    Information Center)
www.pueblo.gsa.gov

International Childbirth
    Education Association (ICEA)
P.O. Box 20048
Minneapolis, MN 55420-0048
(612) 854-8660
www.icea.org

Krames Communications
1100 Grundy Lane
San Bruno, CA 94066-3030
(800) 333-3032
www.krames.com

Lamaze International
1200 19th Street, NW,
    Suite 300
Washington, DC 20036-2422
(202) 857-1128
(800) 368-4404
www.lamaze-childbirth.com

Maternity Center Association
48 East 92nd Street
New York, NY 10128
(212) 777-5000
www.maternity.org

National Association of Parents
    and Professionals for Safe
    Alternatives in Childbirth
    (NAPPSAC)
Route 4 Box 646
Marble Hill, MO 63764
(573) 238-2010
napsac@clas.net

National Family Planning
    and Reproductive Health
    Association
1627 K Street, 12th Floor
Washington, DC 20006
(202) 628-3535
www.nfprha.org

National Health Information
  Center
P.O. Box 1133
Washington, DC 20013
(800) 336-4797
nhic-nt.health.org

National Maternal and Child
  Health Clearinghouse
2070 Chain Bridge Road,
  Suite 450
Vienna, VA 22182-2536
(703) 356-1964
www.nmchc.org

National Women's Health
  Network
514 10th Street, NW
Washington, DC 20004
(202) 347-1140

Parents Without Partners
  International, Inc.
401 North Michigan Avenue
Chicago, IL 60611-4267
(312) 644-6610

(800) 637-7974
www.parentswithoutpartners.org

Planned Parenthood Federation of
  America
810 Seventh Avenue
New York, NY 10019
(212) 261-4300
(800) 829-7732
www.plannedparenthood.org

Single Mothers by Choice
P.O. Box 1642
Gracie Square Station
New York, NY 10028
(212) 988-0993

Single Parent Resource Center
31 East 28th Street
New York, NY 10016
(212) 951-7030
singleparentresources.com

Women in Crisis
360 West 125th Street, Suite 11
New York, NY 10027
(212) 665-2018

Glossary

Abortion—The termination of a pregnancy, either spontaneously by the body or induced through medical intervention prior to the twentieth week of pregnancy.

Abruptio placenta—An emergency situation characterized by the premature separation of the placenta from the uterus.

Adhesions—Scar tissue normally formed by the body following surgery, infection, inflammation, or disease.

Adrenal glands—Endocrine glands above the kidneys that secrete important hormones such as epinephrine and cortisone.

AID—See artificial insemination by donor.

AIH—See artificial insemination by husband.

Alpha fetoprotein (AFP)—A protein normally produced by the fetus's liver but produced in excess in the presence of certain fetal abnormalities.

Amniocentesis—A prenatal procedure in which a small amount of the amniotic fluid that surrounds the fetus is removed for analysis.

Amniotic sac—The sac containing the fetus and the "bag of waters" or amniotic fluid.

Androgen—Male hormone, such as testosterone, produced by the testes and responsible for male characteristics.

Anencephaly—Born without a brain or spinal cord.

Anomaly—A deviation from the normal; malformation.

Anoxia—An abnormal lack of oxygen.

Antenatal—Prior to birth; prenatal.

Antepartal—Prior to labor and delivery.

Antibody—A protein manufactured by the immune system that reacts against specific foreign substances (antigens).

Apnea—The temporary absence of respiration.

Artificial insemination by donor (AID)—A process in which the sperm of a donor male is inseminated into a woman's vagina, cervix, or uterus.

Artificial insemination by husband (AIH)—A process in which a man's sperm is inseminated into his wife's vagina, cervix, or uterus.

Assisted reproductive technology (ART)—All treatments or procedures that involve the handling of human eggs and sperm for the purpose of helping a woman become pregnant. Types of ART include in vitro fertilization, gamete intrafallopian transfer, zygote intrafallopian transfer, embryo cryopreservation, egg or embryo donation, and surrogate birth.

Azoospermia—The absence of sperm during ejaculation.

Bacteriuria—Bacteria in the urine.

Basal body temperature (BBT)—The temperature upon awakening and prior to any activity.

Beta-thalassemia—A type of hereditary anemia occurring in populations bordering the Mediterranean and Southeast Asia.

Betamethasone—A cortisone-like hormone sometimes given to women in premature labor in order to promote fetal lung maturity.

Blighted ovum—An egg that does not develop properly.

Bradycardia—Slower-than-normal heartbeat.

Braxton Hicks contractions—Painless contractions, usually normal.

Breech position—Fetal position in which the buttocks and/or feet are down prior to delivery.

Capacitation—A natural process occurring in sperm after ejaculation that alters the sperm so they can penetrate the egg.

Caudal anesthesia—A type of anesthesia injected into the air spaces around the spinal column that numbs the nerve endings leading to the legs and pelvic area.

Cauterization—The destruction of tissue with an electrical current. Sometimes used to stop bleeding after surgery.

Centrifuge—A device that spins test tubes at high speeds in order to perform special tests on the specimen.

Cephalic—Relating to the head.

Cephalic position—Fetal position where the head is down.

Cerclage—A suture placed around an incompetent cervix to prevent miscarriage; Shirodkar procedure.

Cervical mucus—Normal secretions of the cervix, which change in texture and consistency during different times of the month.

Cervix—The lower end of the uterus, which connects the uterus to the vagina.

Cesarean delivery—The surgical delivery of a baby through an incision made in the mother's abdomen.

Chlamydia—A bacterial sexually transmitted disease.

Chromosome—The part of the nucleus of a body cell that contains a person's genetic material in twisted strands called DNA.

Cleft lip—Congenital fissure of the lip; harelip.

Clomiphene citrate (Clomid)—A commonly used fertility drug that induces ovulation.

Conception—The impregnation of a female ovum by the male's sperm to create a new being.

Congenital—Born with; existing before or from birth.

Corpus luteum—A body formed on the ovary following ovulation, which secretes progesterone to prepare the body for pregnancy.

Cranium—The part of the skull enclosing the brain.

Crowning—The appearance of the baby's head at the entrance of the vagina during delivery.

Culture—Laboratory test to detect the growth of certain microorganisms that might be causing an infection.

Danazol (Danocrine)—A drug used to treat endometriosis.

D&C—See dilation and curettage.

Diethylstilbestrol (DES)—A synthetic estrogen used between 1940 and 1970 to prevent miscarriage. Has been related to congenital abnormalities in the offspring.

Dilation and curettage (D&C)—A procedure in which the interior of the uterus is scraped to diagnose a disease, empty uterine contents, or correct vaginal bleeding.

Dysmenorrhea—Painful menstruation.

Dystocia—Abnormal labor.

Eclampsia—Severe hypertension of pregnancy, sometimes accompanied by coma and convulsions.

Ectopic pregnancy—A pregnancy outside the inner lining of the uterus, such as in a fallopian tube, the abdomen, the cervix, or an ovary.

Effacement—The thinning and shortening of the cervix during labor.

Ejaculation—The emission of semen from the male urethra during climax.

Embryo—The name given to the product of conception from the time of implantation until the eighth week. It is then called the fetus.

Endometriosis—The abnormal growth of endometrial tissue outside the uterus.

Endometrium—The inner membrane lining of the uterus.

Epididymis—The duct system responsible for sperm maturation and their ability to fertilize an egg; responsible for sperm transfer.

Episiotomy—An incision made in the perineum during delivery to prevent lacerations and to facilitate delivery.

Erythroblastosis fetalis—A type of newborn anemia due to mother-
child blood-incompatibility problems.

Estriol—A form of estrogen that increases during pregnancy.

Estrogen—A female hormone responsible for female secondary sex traits.

Fallopian tubes—A pair of tubes that retrieve and carry the eggs from
the ovaries to the uterus for implantation; fertilization occurs here.

Fertility—Capability to reproduce and to bear offspring.

Fertilization—The union of the egg and the sperm marking the beginning of pregnancy.

Fetal distress—A critical condition of the fetus, usually during labor, in
which the fetus's life may be in jeopardy.

Fetus—Product of conception from the eighth week of gestation until
birth.

Follicle-stimulating hormone (FSH)—Hormone released by the pituitary gland that triggers ovum development or sperm production.

Forceps—Metal device that is sometimes used during delivery to protect
the baby's head and assist it through the birth canal.

Fructose—Produced by the seminal vesicles; the sugar that sperm use
for energy.

FSH—See follicle-stimulating hormone.

Fundus—The upper, rounded, muscular, and contracting part of the uterus.

Gamete—A sexual cell; unfertilized egg or mature sperm cell.

Gamete intrafallopian tube transfer (GIFT)—A procedure in which one
or more eggs from the woman's ovaries are removed, mixed with
sperm, and then placed in the fallopian tube(s) for fertilization.

Gene—The hereditary factor in a chromosome that carries characteristics from one generation to another.

General anesthesia—A type of anesthesia that induces unconsciousness.

Gestational diabetes—Diabetes that occurs only during pregnancy.

GIFT—See gamete intrafallopian tube transfer.

Glomeronephritis—A serious type of kidney infection.

GnRH—See gonadotropin-releasing hormone.

Gonads—The ovaries or testes.

Gonadotropin-releasing hormone (GnRH)—A hormone secreted by
the hypothalamus that stimulates the pituitary to release FSH and
LH hormones.

Gonorrhea—A sexually transmitted disease caused by a bacteria.

Gynecologist—A physician specializing in female reproduction, pregnancy, and often birth.

Habitual aborter—A woman who has miscarried three or more times.

Hamster test—A test of the ability of a man's sperm to penetrate a hamster egg stripped of its outer membrane.

Harelip—See cleft lip.

hCG—See human chorionic gonadotropin.

High-risk pregnancy—A pregnancy in which there is a chance of a problem developing that might jeopardize the life or health of mother and/or baby.

hMG—See human menopausal gonadotropin.

Hormone—A chemical substance secreted by an organ that initiates or regulates activity in another part of the body.

HSG—See hysterosalpingogram.

Hühner test—A test that assesses the quantity and quality of cervical mucus and how the sperm react to it; postcoital test.

Humagon—The luteinizing and follicle-stimulating hormones recovered from the urine of postmenopausal women that is used to induce multiple ovulation in various fertility treatments.

Human chorionic gonadotropin (hCG)—A hormone produced by the placenta early in pregnancy; used as the basis of pregnancy tests.

Human menopausal gonadotropin (hMG)—A fertility drug derived from the urine of postmenopausal women; Humagon.

Hyaline membrane disease—A lung disorder of premature infants caused by lack of surfactant production; respiratory distress syndrome.

Hydatiform mole—A cancer of the placenta.

Hydramnios—Excessive amniotic fluid.

Hydrocephalus—Excessive fluid in the skull.

Hyperglycemia—High blood sugar.

Hypoglycemia—Low blood sugar.

Hypoxia—Insufficient amount of oxygen.

Hysterectomy—The removal of the uterus.

Hysterosalpingogram (HSG)—An X-ray done in the infertility investigation in which dye is injected to view the female anatomy.

Implantation—The attachment of the fertilized ovum in the uterus.

Impotence—A man's inability to have an erection and/or ejaculate.

Incompetent cervix—The inability of the cervix to remain closed during pregnancy, resulting in spontaneous abortion.

Incomplete abortion—A miscarriage in which some tissue has passed but some remains in the uterus.

Induction—The process of causing or producing, as in the induction of labor with drugs to stimulate uterine contractions.

Infertility—The inability to conceive after one year of unprotected intercourse.

Intrauterine device (IUD)—A device placed in the uterus as a means of contraception.

Intrauterine growth retardation (IUGR)—A reduction in fetal growth for reasons such as infection, inadequate placenta, or exposure to teratogens.

Intrauterine transfusion—A procedure in which blood is introduced into the fetus's abdomen; used for severe maternal-fetal blood incompatibilities.

In vitro fertilization (IVF)—A process in which eggs are extracted from a woman and fertilized with a man's sperm, and the embryo is transferred to the uterus for development.

IUGR—See intrauterine growth retardation.

IUD—See intrauterine device.

IVF—See in vitro fertilization.

Jaundice—Yellow discoloration of the skin due to elevated bilirubin (formed from the breakdown of red blood cells).

Kegel exercises—Exercises for the muscles surrounding the vagina.

Labor—The process of giving birth, divided into three stages ending with complete cervical dilation, delivery, and the expulsion of the placenta.

Lactation—The act of giving milk.

Laparoscopy—A surgical procedure in which a small telescope is inserted beside the navel to view the female reproductive organs.

Laparotomy—An incision made in the abdomen.

Lecithin/sphingomyelin ratio (LS ratio)—A chemical test on the amniotic fluid to detect fetal lung maturity.

LH hormone—See luteinizing hormone.

Low forceps—Forceps applied during delivery after the fetal head is showing.

L/S ratio—See lecithin/sphingomyelin ratio.

Luteal phase—The time from ovulation to menstruation.

Luteal-phase defect—A short luteal phase characterized by inadequate progesterone production.

Luteinizing hormone (LH)—A pituitary hormone that stimulates the secretion of progesterone in women and testosterone production in men.

Magnesium sulfate—A medication used to treat toxemia and sometimes to prevent premature labor.

Malpresentation—Abnormal fetal position.

Meconium—The first feces of a newborn infant. If seen during pregnancy, it usually indicates fetal distress.

Menstrual cycle—The monthly menstruation cycle starting with the first day of menses and ending on the first day of the next menses. Ranges from twenty-five to thirty-five days.

Menstruation—The shedding of the endometrium when pregnancy does not occur.

Midwife—A person who delivers infants. A certified nurse-midwife is a registered nurse who has graduated from a nurse-midwifery program and has taken a certifying exam.

Miscarriage—A pregnancy loss prior to the twentieth week, most often in the first trimester; spontaneous abortion.

Missed abortion—A miscarriage whereby bleeding occurs and the baby dies, but it is not naturally expelled and must be removed by a D&C.

Molding—The process in which the fetal head changes to fit the pelvis during labor.

Neonatal—Pertaining to the first four weeks of life.

Neonatal death—Death occurring during the first four weeks of life.

Neonatology—The field of pediatrics concerned with the care of newborn infants. Often pertains to high-risk newborns.

Neural tube defects—A group of malformations caused by abnormal development of the nervous system.

Nonstress test (NST)—A test assessing fetal heart rate and its response to spontaneous movements or contractions.

Nullipara—A woman who has not borne children.

Obstetrician—A physician who specializes in female reproduction, pregnancy, and birth.

OCT—See oxytocin challenge test.

Oligohydramnios—Inadequate amount of amniotic fluid.

Oligospermia—An inadequate sperm count.

OT—See ovum transfer.

Ovary—One of a pair of female reproductive organs that stores and releases eggs with ovulation and secretes hormones such as estrogen and progesterone.

Oviduct—A fallopian tube.

Ovulation—The release of an egg from an ovary.

Ovum transfer (OT)—The transfer of a fertilized egg from a donor's to a recipient woman's uterus.

Oxytocin—A hormone that stimulates uterine contractions.

Oxytocin challenge test (OCT)—A test of fetal well-being in which the mother is given small amounts of oxytocin and the fetal heart rate is monitored.

Pap smear—A slide analysis of cervical cells for abnormalities.

Pelvic inflammatory disease (PID)—Inflammation of the pelvic organs, especially caused by bacterial infection.

Parlodel—A drug that reduces levels of the pituitary hormone prolactin.

Perinatal—Before, during, and immediately after birth.

Perinatology—Specialty of obstetrics dealing with the care of high-risk mothers and their babies; maternal-fetal medicine.

Perineum—The area between the vagina and the rectum.

Phenylketonuria (PKU)—A hereditary deficiency of the liver enzyme needed to convert phenylalanine into a usable form.

PID—See pelvic inflammatory disease.

Pitocin—A synthetic form of oxytocin.

Pituitary gland—The master endocrine gland located at the base of the brain; secretes various hormones and oversees complex chemical interactions.

Placenta—A vascular organ in the pregnant uterus from which the fetus receives its nourishment; forms the communication between mother and child.

Placenta previa—Placenta implanted in the lower part of the uterus so that it partially or totally covers the cervical opening.

Polycystic kidney disease—An inherited disease characterized by cysts on the kidney causing the kidney to enlarge.

Polycystic ovarian syndrome—A hormone problem in which ovulation fails to occur and instead small cysts form in the ovaries; Stein-Leventhal syndrome.

Polyhydramnios—Excessive amniotic fluid.

Postcoital test—See Hühner test.

Postmaturity—Pregnancy continuing after the fortieth week.

Postnatal—Occurring after birth.

Postterm—A fetus of a gestational age over forty-two weeks; postmature.

Preeclampsia—A hypertensive disorder of pregnancy without seizures or coma.

Premature—Born after the twentieth week and prior to the thirty-seventh week of gestation.

Presentation—The position of the baby in the uterus.

Preterm—See premature.

Primigravida—A woman who is pregnant for the first time.

Progesterone—A hormone responsible for preparing the uterus for implantation. Secreted by the placenta during pregnancy.

Progestin—See progesterone.

Prolactin—The pituitary hormone that in high amounts stimulates milk production.

Prostaglandins—Hormones used to induce labor.

Prostate gland—A male gland near the bladder that contributes to ejaculation fluid; it is prone to infections that may affect male fertility.

Proteinuria—The presence of protein in the urine.

Pudendal nerve block—Local anesthetic given into the pudendal nerves on both sides of the perineum.

Quickening—Fetal movement perceived by the mother.

Radioimmunoassay—A pregnancy test measuring antigen-antibody reaction with a radioisotope technique.

Respiratory distress syndrome (RDS)—See hyaline membrane disease.

Retrolental fibroplasia—A condition caused by high oxygen concentration given to premature infants; results in blindness.

Rh factor—An antigenic substance present in the red blood cells of most people; those having the factor are called Rh-positive and those who do not are called Rh-negative.

RhoGam—An immunizing agent given to Rh-negative women following birth to prevent production of antibodies in any Rh-positive babies they may have in the future.

Rubella—German measles.

Rubin's test—A procedure testing tubal patency; rare today; replaced by hysterosalpingogram.

Saddle block—Local anesthetic in the dura sac (outer membrane covering the spinal cord) that numbs the pelvic area.

Semen—The thick, cloudy secretion containing sperm discharged from the male urethra during sexual excitement; seminal fluid.

Semen analysis—The laboratory examination of semen to check the quality and quantity of sperm.

Seminal fluid—See semen.

Septate uterus—A congenital abnormality whereby the uterus is divided into two compartments.

Sexually transmitted disease (STD)—Any disease or infection transmitted through sexual contact through the genitals, mouth, or anus; venereal disease.

SGA—See small for gestational age.

Shirodkar procedure—See cerclage.

Sickle-cell—A hereditary type of anemia caused by malformed red blood cells.

Small for gestational age (SGA)—A baby who weighs less than 90 percent of the average infant at the same stage of pregnancy or delivery.

Sperm—Male germ cell produced by the testicle.

Sperm count—The number of sperm in the male's ejaculate.

Sperm washing—A laboratory technique that separates the sperm from the seminal fluid.

Spermatic cord—The cord suspending the testes. It is composed of veins, arteries, lymphatics, nerves, and the vas deferens.

Spinal anesthesia—Anesthesia injected into the spine to produce numbness below the waist.

Spontaneous abortion—See miscarriage.

STD—See sexually transmitted disease.

Stein-Leventhal syndrome—See polycystic ovarian syndrome.

Sterility—The inability to produce children; untreatable infertility.

Stillborn—The death of a fetus before or during delivery.

Stress test—A now rare method of detecting fetal well-being by monitoring its response to contractions induced with oxytocin.

Surfactant—A substance produced in the fetal lung necessary for lung maturity.

Surrogate mother—A woman who brings to term a couple's biological child, often as stipulated in a contract.

Synarel—A synthetic hormone used to treat endometriosis.

Syndrome—A complex of signs and symptoms resulting in a specific clinical picture of a disease or abnormality.

Syphilis—A sexually transmitted disease caused by a bacteria.

Tay-Sachs—A congenital disease affecting the fat metabolism and the brain. Symptoms include progressive weakness, disability, blindness, and finally death.

Teratogen—Any substance capable of causing malformations in a developing embryo.

Testicular biopsy—Inspection of a small piece of testicular tissue under a microscope.

Testosterone—Hormone produced by the testicles that is responsible for male sex characteristics.

Threatened abortion—Bleeding prior to the twentieth week of pregnancy.

Thrombophlebitis—Inflammation of a vein.

Thyroid—A gland situated in the front of the neck that is essential to normal growth and metabolic processes.

TORCH organisms—Toxoplasmosis, syphilis, rubella, cytomegalovirus, herpes simplex, and other diseases that may harm the embryo/fetus.

Toxemia—Hypertension during pregnancy.

Trimester—Three-month period during pregnancy; there are three trimesters during pregnancy.

Tubal patency—Open fallopian tubes.

Tubal pregnancy—Pregnancy occurring in a fallopian tube.

Ultrasound—A test in which high-frequency sound waves are used to detect fetal well-being and diagnose defects.

Undescended testicles—Testes that fail to descend into the scrotum during fetal development.

UPI—See uteroplacental insufficiency.

Urologist—A physician specializing in the male reproductive system and urinary-tract diseases in both men and women.

Uterine fibroids—Benign tumors on the outside, inside, or within the wall of the uterus, often changing the size and shape of the uterus.

Uterus—The female reproductive organ responsible for bearing the fetus from implantation until birth; womb.

Uteroplacental insufficiency (UPI)—Condition in which the placenta is unable to meet the oxygen and nutritional needs of the developing fetus.

Vagina—The muscular passage from the uterus to the outside of the body.

Varicocele—An enlargement of the vein of the spermatic cord.

Vas deferens—Two tubes that extend from the epidermis to the prostate; carry sperm from the epididymis to the ejaculatory duct.

Vasography—An X-ray study of the vas deferens.

Venereal disease—See sexually transmitted disease.

Version—A procedure in which the fetus and uterus are manipulated in order to turn the fetus to a "head-down" position.

Vertex—Top of head.

Viable—Capable of sustaining life; after twenty-eight weeks of gestation.

Womb—See uterus.

X-linked inheritance—Inheritance through genes located on the X chromosome.

Zona pellucida—The protective coating surrounding the egg.

Zygote—The developing ovum from the time of fertilization until implantation in the uterus.

Bibliography

Aaronson, L. S., and C. L. Macnee (1989). "Tobacco, Alcohol and Caffeine Use During Pregnancy." *Journal of Gynecological and Neonatal Nursing* July/August, pp. 279–285.

American Association of Critical-Care Nurses (1983). "High Risk Neonatal Nursing." In Vestal, K. W., and C.A.M. McKenzie, eds., *Perinatal Nursing*. Philadelphia: W. B. Saunders.

American College of Gynecologists and Obstetricians (1984). Women's Health Series: *Exercise and Fitness*.

American College of Gynecologists and Obstetricians (1988). *Guidelines for Vaginal Delivery After a Previous Cesarean Birth*.

Andrews, L. B. (1985). *New Conceptions*. New York: Ballantine Books.

Arias, F. (1984). *High-Risk Pregnancy and Delivery*. St. Louis, MO: C. V. Mosby.

Asch, R., J. Balmaceda, L. Ellsworth, and P. Wong (1985). "Gamete Intra-fallopian Transfer (GIFT): New Treatment for Infertility." *International Journal of Fertility* 30(1), pp. 41–45.

Beck, W. W. Jr., and E. E. Wallach (1981). "When Therapy Fails—Artificial Insemination." *Contemporary OB/GYN* 17, p. 113.

Beckman, D. A., and R. L. Brent (1986). "Mechanism of Known Environmental Teratogens: Drugs and Chemicals." *Clinical Perontology* 13, pp. 649–87.

Bellina, J. H., and J. Wilson (1985). *You Can Have a Baby*. New York: Crown.

Berger, G. S. (1989). *The Couple's Guide to Fertility*. New York: Doubleday.

Berkowitz, G. S. (1986). "Epidemiology of Infertility and Early Pregnancy Wastage." In Alan H. DeCherney, ed., *Reproductive Failure*, pp. 17–20. New York: Churchill Livingstone.

——— (1990). "Delayed Childbearing and the Outcome of Pregnancy." *The New England Journal of Medicine* 322(10), pp. 659–664.

Billingsley, J. (1980). "The Child Who Never Arrived: A New Look at Miscarriage." *Ladies Home Journal* November, pp. 33–38.

Bills, B. (1980). "Nursing Considerations: Administering Labor-Suppressing Medications." *Maternal Child Nursing*, pp. 252–256.

Blackburn, S., and L. Lowen (1986). "Impact of an Infant's Premature Birth on the Grandparents and Parents." *Journal of Obstetric, Gynecologic, and Neonatal Nursing*, pp. 173–178.

Blakemore, K., and M. Mahoney (1986). "Chorionic Villus Sampling." In A. Milunsky, ed., *Genetics and the Fetus*, pp. 625–655. New York: Plenum Press.

Bobak, Irene, et al. (1989). *Maternity and Gynecologic Care*. St. Louis, MO: C.V. Mosby.

Boggs, K. R., and P. K. Rau (1983). "Breast-Feeding the Premature Infant." *American Journal of Nursing*, pp. 1437–1439.

Borg, S., and J. Lasker (1981). *When Pregnancy Fails*. Boston: Beacon Press.

Boutelle, A. (1978). "Suspense in Pregnancy." *Vogue* September, pp. 307–312.

Brackbill, Y., and D. Young (1984). *Birth Trap*. New York: Warner Books.

Brengman, S., and M. Burns (1983). "Vaginal Delivery After C-section." *The American Journal of Nursing* November, pp. 1544–1547.

Brewer, G. S., and T. Brewer (1985). *The Truth About Diet and Drugs in Pregnancy: What Every Pregnant Woman Should Know*. New York: Penguin Books.

Brown, M. J., D. Bellinger, and J. Matthews (1990). "In Utero Lead Exposure." *Maternal Child Nursing* March/April, 15, pp. 94.

Brown, V. (1987). "Male Infertility." *Postgraduate Medicine* 81(2), pp. 217–219.

Brucker, M. C., and N. J. Macmullen, (1985). "What's New in Pregnancy Tests." *Journal of Obstetric, Gynecologic and Neonatal Nursing*, pp. 353–359.

Burke, R. K., and L. Kapinos (1985). "The Effect of In Vitro Sperm Capacitation on Sperm Velocity and Motility As Measured by an In-Office, Integrated Microcomputerized System for Semen Analysis." *International Journal of Fertility* 30(2), pp. 10–18.

Campbell, B. (1986). "Overdue Delivery: Its Impact on Mothers-to-Be." *Maternal Child Nursing* 11, pp. 170–172.

Canadian Foundation for the Study of Infant Deaths (1991). *Information About Sudden Infant Death Syndrome*. Toronto, Canada: Canadian Foundation for the Study of Infant Deaths.

Charlish, A., and L. H. Holt (1991). *Birth-Tech: Tests and Technology in Pregnancy and Birth*. New York: Facts on File.

Chism, Denise (1998). *The High-Risk Pregnancy Sourcebook*. L.A.: Lowell House.

Cole, K. C. (1980). *What Only a Mother Can Tell You About Having a Baby*. New York: Berkeley Books.

Collins, C. (1987). "Gestational Diabetes." *American Baby* June, pp. 45–46.

Cook, P. "Drugs and Pregnancy." New York: The American Council for Drug Education. Congress Catalog Card Number: 86–070944.

Cox News Service (1991). "One-Year Study Will Involve Testing Georgia Newborns for Cocaine." *Orlando Sentinel* Thursday, March 14, p. A6.

Crout, T. K. (1980). "Caring for the Mother of a Stillborn Baby." *Nursing* 10(4), April, pp. 70–73.

D'Amica, J. F., and J. C. Gambone (1989). "Advances in the Management of the Infertile Couple." *Advances in Fertility Practice* 39(5), pp. 257–264.

Davis, L. (1987). "Daily Fetal Movement Counting." *Journal of Nurse-Midwifery* 32(1), pp. 11–19.

Demarest, C. B., ed. (1985). "CC: I Can't Get Pregnant." *Patient Care* November 15, pp. 97–119.

DeVita, V., S. Hellman, and S. Rosenberg (1986). *AIDS: Etiology, Diagnosis, Treatment and Prevention*. Philadelphia: J. B. Lippincott.

Dorris, M. (1989). *The Broken Cord*. New York: Harper & Row.

Dowsett, C. A. (1984). "Sudden Infant Death Syndrome." *Ladycom* November/December, pp. 21–24.

Elias, S., and Annas, G. J. (1987). "Fetal and Gene Therapy." *Current Problems in Obstetrics, Gynecology and Fertility* 10(3).

Elmer-Dewitt, P. (1990). "A Revolution in Making Babies." *Time* November 5, pp. 76–77.

Epiro, P., ed. (1984). "When Sudden Infant Death Strikes." *Patient Care* March, 15, pp. 18–42.

Federal-Provincial Subcommittee on Nutrition (1987). *Nutrition in Pregnancy: National Guidelines*. Ottawa, Canada: Health and Welfare Canada.

Freeman, E. W. (1984–1985). "Emotional Needs of Infertile Couples." *Current Therapy of Infertility*, pp. 268–271.

Freeman, R., and Pescar, S. (1982). *Safe Delivery*. New York: McGraw Hill.

Garner, H. H. (1983). "In Vitro Fertilization and Embryo Transfer." *Journal of Obstetrics, Gynecology and Neonatal Nursing* April, pp. 75–78.

Garner, M. (1987). "Miracle Babies: The Next Generation." *Self* June, pp. 129–133.

Gilbert, E. S., and J. S. Harmon (1986). *High-Risk Pregnancy and Delivery: Nursing Perspectives*. St. Louis, MO: C. V. Mosby.

Gindoff, P. R., and R. Jewelewicz (1986). "Reproductive Potential in Older Women." *Fertility and Sterility* 46(6), pp. 898–1001.

Goldberg, J. (1991). "Can They Save This Baby?" *Reader's Digest* January, pp. 1–15.

Gonzalez, E. R. (1983). "Sperm Swim Singly After Vitamin C Therapy." *Journal of American Medical Association* 49(20), pp. 2747–2751.

Govani, L. E., and J. E. Hayes, (1985). *Drugs and Nursing Implications*. Norwalk, CT: Appleton-Century-Crofts.

Griffin, M. E. (1983). "Resolving Infertility: An Emotional Crisis." *Association of Operating Room Nurses Journal* 38(4), pp. 597–601.

Gwinn, Marta, et al. (1991). "Prevalence of HIV Infection in Childbearing Women in the United States." *The Journal of the American Medical Association* 265(13), pp. 1704–1708.

Hales, D., and R. K. Creasy (1982). *New Hope for Problem Pregnancies*. New York: Berkley Books.

Harkness, C. (1987). *The Infertility Book*. Volcano, California: Volcano Press.

Harrison, L. L., and S. Twardosz (1986). "Teaching Mothers About Their Preterm Infants." *Journal of Obstetric, Gynecologic, and Neonatal Nursing* March/April, 15(2), pp. 165–172.

Harrison, M., M. Golbus, and R. Filly (1984). *The Unborn Patient: Prenatal Diagnosis and Treatment*. Orlando, FL: Grune & Stratton.

Hemmer, M., M. Staquet, and A. Baert, eds. (1986). *Clinical Aspects of AIDS and AIDS-Related Complex*. Oxford: Oxford University Press.

Hillard, P.A. (1984). "Twins." *Parents* December, pp. 142–144.

Huggins, G. (1988). Interview with author. February.

——— (1990). "When Your Baby Is Breech." *Parents* September, pp. 150–151.

Ilse, S. (1985). *Empty Arms: Coping After Miscarriage, Stillbirth and Infant Death*. Maple Plain, Minnesota: Wintergreen Press.

International Childbirth Education Association. "Smoking and Childbearing: Maternal and Fetal Complications." *International Journal of Childbirth Education* 10(2), pp. IR–7R.

Jason, Janine, and A. Van Der Mer (1989). *Parenting Your Premature Baby*. New York: Henry Holt.

Jensen, M. D., R. Benson, and I. Bobak (1977). *Maternity Care: The Nurse and the Family*. St. Louis, MO: C. V. Mosby.

Johnson, J., et al. (1986). *Trying to Conceive*. Omaha, NE: Centering Corporation.

Kinney, J. M. (1984). "Pediatric Surgeons Focus on Congenital Defects." *Association of Operating Room Nurses Journal* 39(2), pp. 195–196.

Kitzinger, S. (1985). *Birth over Thirty*. Toronto: Penguin.

Klaus, M. H., and J. H. Kennell (1982). *Parent-Infant Bonding*. St. Louis, MO: C. V. Mosby.

Knight, B. (1983). *Sudden Death in Infants: The Cot Syndrome*. London: Penguin.

Knuppel, R. A., and Drukker, J. (1986). *High-Risk Pregnancy: A Team Approach*. Philadelphia: W. B. Saunders.

Kredentser, J. V. (1986). "Infertility: A Review of Physical and Emotional Aspects." *Canadian Family Physician* 32, pp. 1651–1655.

Laberge, J. M. (1986). "Fetal Surgery: Considering the Fetus as Patient." *Canadian Family Physician* 32, pp. 2099–2103.

LaCerva, V. (1981). *Breast-Feeding: A Manual for Health Professionals*. Garden City, NJ: Medical Examination Publishing.

Lauersen, N. H. (1983). *Childbirth with Love*. New York: Berkley Books.

Liebman, B. (1987). "Eating for Two." *Nutrition Action Health Letter* 14(3), pp. 1–4.

Linn, S., et al. (1982). "Delay in Conception for Former 'Pill' Users." *Journal of American Medical Association* 247(5), pp. 629–632.

Lipsultz, L. I., and Serono Symposia, USA (1989). *Male Infertility*. Norwell, MA: Serono Symposia.

Lynch, M., and V. A. McKeon (1990). "Cocaine Use During Pregnancy: Research Findings and Clinical Implications." *Journal of Gynecological and Neonatal Nursing* July/August 19(4), pp. 285–291.

McDonald-Grandin, M. (1983). *Will I Ever Be a Mother?* Portland, Oregon: Celeste Books.

McNally, M. (1987). "Male Infertility: 3 Endocrine Causes." *Postgraduate Medicine* 81 (2), pp. 207–213.

March of Dimes Birth Defects (1987). *Counseling*. White Plains, N.Y.

Marlow, D. (1977). *Textbook of Pediatric Nursing*. Philadelphia: W. B. Saunders.

Marmet, C. (1981). *Manual Expression of Breast Milk: Marmet Technique*. Pamphlet No. 107. Franklin Park, IL: La Leche League.

Martel, S., A. Wacholder, A. Lippman, J. Broham, and E. Hamilton (1987). "Maternal Age and Primary Cesarean Rates: A Multivariate Analysis." *American Journal of Obstetrics and Gynecology* 156(2), pp. 305–308.

Melis, G. B., et al. (1987). "Pharmacological Induction of Multiple Follicular Development Improves the Success Rate of Artificial Insemination with Husband's Sperm in Couples with Male-Related or Unexplained Infertility." *Fertility and Sterility* 47(3), pp. 441–445.

Michaels, E. (1985). "Inducing Labor in Pregnant Women." *Chatelaine* February, p. 18.

Mills, J. L., B. L. Graubard, E. E. Harley, et al. (1984). "Maternal Alcohol Consumption and Birthweight: How Much Drinking During Pregnancy Is Safe?" *Journal of American Medical Association* 252(14), pp. 1875–1879.

Milunsky, A. (1986). *Genetic Disorders and the Fetus.* New York: Plenum Press.

Moore, K. A. (1990). *Facts at a Glance.* November. Washington, DC: Child Trends Inc.

Moore, M. L. (1983). *Realities in Childbearing.* Philadelphia: W. B. Saunders.
———— (1989). "Recurrent Teen Pregnancy: Making it Less Desirable." *Maternal Child Nursing* 14, March/April, pp. 104–109.

Naeye, R. L. (1979). "Coitus and Associated Amniotic Fluid Infection." *New England Journal of Medicine* 301, p. 1198.

Nance, S. (1982). *Premature Babies.* New York: Berkley Books.

National Center for Health Statistics (1986). *Monthly Vital Statistics.* September 26. Washington, D.C.

Newsweek (1990). "Making Babies After Menopause." *Newsweek* November 5, p. 76.

Nofzinger, M. (1982). *The Fertility Question.* Tennessee: The Book Publishing Co.

Nursing Photobook (1982). *Attending OB/GYN Patients.* Pennsylvania: Intermed Communications.

Office Technology Education Project (n.d.). *VDT's, Radiation and Pregnancy.* Somerville, MA: Office Technology Education Project.

Olin, B., ed. (1991). *Facts and Comparisons,* Inc. St. Louis, MO.

Osofsy, H., and Drukker, J. (1986). "Sexual Intimacy in Pregnancy." In Knuppel, R. A., and I. E. Drukker, eds., *High-Risk Pregnancy: A Team Approach.* Philadelphia: W. B. Saunders, pp.187–199.

Palinski, C., and H. Pfizer (1980). *Coping with Miscarriage.* New York: New American Library.

Pletch, P. K. (1990). "Birth Defect Prevention: Nursing Interventions." *Journal of Gynecological and Neonatal Nursing* 19(6), November/December, pp. 482–487.

Public Health Education Information Sheet (1985). "PKU." White Plains, NY: March of Dimes Birth Defects Foundation.

Public Health Education Information Sheet (1986). "Tay-Sachs." White Plains, NY: March of Dimes Birth Defects Foundation.

Purvis, A. (1990). "Major Surgery Before Birth Time." *Time* June 11, p. 55.

Quindlen, A. (1987). "Baby Craving." *Life* June, pp. 33–34.

Rapp, R. (1984). "The Ethics of Choice." *Ms. Magazine* April, pp. 97–100.

Redshaw, M. E., R. P. Rivers, and D. B. Rosenblatt (1985). *Born Too Early*. London: Oxford.

Resolve, Inc. (1986). *The Emotional Impact of Miscarriage*. Belmont, MA: Resolve, Inc.

———. (1986). *Medical Causes of Miscarriage*. Belmont, MA: Resolve, Inc.

Reynolds, J. L. (1986). "Prenatal Diagnosis by Amniocentesis and Chorionic Villus Biopsy." *Canadian Family Physician* 32, pp. 105–108.

Riccardi, V. (1977). *The Genetic Approach to Human Disease*. New York: Oxford University Press.

Roberts, F., and M. E. Pembrey (1985). *An Introduction to Medical Genetics*. Oxford: Oxford University Press.

Roberts-Worthington, B., J. Vermeersch, and S. R. Williams (1981). *Nutrition in Pregnancy and Lactation*. St. Louis, MO: C. V. Mosby.

Rodriquez, M. H., et al. (1990). "Comparison of TestPak and Ovustick for Predicting Ovulation." *Journal of Reproductive Medicine* February, pp. 133–135.

Sala, D. J., and K. J. Moise (1990). "The Treatment of Preterm Labor Using a Portable Subcutaneous Terbutaline Pump." *The Journal of Gynecological and Neonatal Nursing* 19(2), March/April, pp. 108–115.

Schwartz, B., et al. (1981). "Exercise-Associated Amenorrhea: A Distinct Entity?" *American Journal of Obstetrics and Gynecology* 15, pp. 662–670.

Schwiebert, P., and P. Kirk (1985). *When Hello Means Goodbye*. Portland, OR: Perinatal Loss.

Seligmann, J., and L. Wilson (1990). "The Tiniest Patients." *Newsweek* June 11, pp. 56–57.

Sherman, K., J. Daling, and N. Weiss (1987). "Sexually Transmitted Diseases and Tubal Infertility." *Sexually Transmitted Diseases* January/March, 14(1), pp. 12–16.

Shettles, L. B., and Rorvik, D. M. (1984). *How to Choose the Sex of Your Baby*. New York: Doubleday.

Shortridge, L. A. (1983). "Using Ritodrine Hydrochloride to Inhibit Preterm Labor." *Maternal Child Nursing* January/February, 8(1), pp. 58–61.

Shosenberg, N. (1980). *The Premature Infant: A Handbook for Parents*. Toronto: The Hospital for Sick Children.

Silber, S. J. (1991). *How to Get Pregnant with the New Technology*. New York: Warner Books.

Simkin, P., P. J. Whalley, and A. Keppler (1984). *Pregnancy, Childbirth, and the Newborn*. Deephoven, Minnesota: Meadowbrook Books.

Smith, J. (1988). "The Dangers of Prenatal Cocaine Use." *Maternal Child Nursing* May/June, 13, pp. 174–179.

Squires, S. (1990). "A Cure for Killer Pregnancies." *Ladies Home Journal* October, p. 132.

Stenchever, M. A. (1983). "Habitual Abortion." *Contemporary OB/GYN* 21(1), p. 162.

Stevens, K. A. (1989). "Individualized Prenatal Nursing Care of Pregnant Adolescents Makes a Difference." *Gynecological and Neonatal Nursing* November/December, pp. 521–522.

Suarez, G., R. Swartz, and N. Baum (1987). "Male Infertility." *Postgraduate Medicine* February 1, pp. 203–206.

Thompson, J. M., et al. (1986). *Clinical Nursing*. St. Louis, MO: C. V. Mosby.

Twomey, J. G. (1989). "The Ethics of In Utero Fetal Surgery." *Nursing Clinics of North America* 24(4), December, pp. 1025–31.

Tyckoson, D. A. (1986). *Test Tube Babies: In Vitro Fertilization and Embryo Transfer*. Phoenix, Arizona: Oryx Press.

UCI-AMI Center for Reproductive Health (n.d.). *Your Guide to the UCI-AMI Center for Reproductive Health*.

United States Department of Health and Human Services (1984–85). *Rubella and Congenital Rubella Syndrome*. Washington, D.C.

———— (1990). Aids in Women—United States, as seen in Morbidity Mortality Weekly Report, November 30, 39(47), pp. 845–846.

Urdang, L., and H. H. Swallow (1983). *Mosby's Medical and Nursing Dictionary*. St. Louis, MO: C. V. Mosby.

Utian, W., et al. (1985). "Successful Pregnancy after In Vitro Fertilization and Embryo Transfer from an Infertile Woman to a Surrogate." *The New England Journal of Medicine* 313(21), pp. 1351-2.

Vento, M. (1991). "Where We Stand." *Health Watch* March/April, pp. 49–56.

Williams, M. (1986). "Long-Term Hospitalization of Women with High-Risk Pregnancies." *Journal of Gynecological and Neonatal Nursing* January/February, 15(1), pp. 17–21.

Wilson, B. A. (1991). "The Disease that Cries Wolf." *Health Watch* March/April, pp. 59–63.

Winslow, W. (1987). "First Pregnancy After 35: What Is the Experience?" *Maternal Child Nursing* March/April, 12(2), pp. 92–96.

Wisniewski, L., and K. Hirschorn (1980). *A Guide to Human Chromosome Defects*. White Plains, NY: March of Dimes Birth Defects Foundation.

Index